THE HEALTH OF POULTRY

LONGMAN VETERINARY HEALTH SERIES

Published titles

The Health of Horses
Edited by David G Powell & Stephen G Jackson

Livestock Health and Welfare
Edited by Roy Moss

Forthcoming titles

Small Ruminant Health
Edited by Tony J Wilsmore & Peter J Goddard

Animal Breeding and Infertility
Edited by Michael C Meredith

The Health of Dairy Cattle
Edited by David G White

The Health of Pigs
Edited by John R Hill & David W B Sainsbury

Food Hygiene
Edited by Jeremy Hall

Nutrition and Animal Health
Edited by John T Abrams

THE HEALTH OF POULTRY

Edited by
Mark Pattison

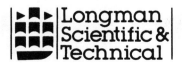

Longman
Scientific &
Technical

Longman Scientific & Technical,
Longman Group UK Limited,
Longman House, Burnt Mill, Harlow,
Essex CM20 2JE, England
and Associated Companies throughout the world.

First published 1993

ISBN 0-582-06579-8

British Library Cataloguing in Publication Data
A CIP record for this book is available from the British Library

Typeset in 10/12½pt Plantin roman by 3MM.

DEDICATION

This book is dedicated to the memory of Cliff Stuart, who died suddenly very soon after completing the turkey chapter for this book. He was always an inspiration to his veterinary colleagues concerned with poultry medicine combining cheerful common-sense with an incisive intellect and an ability to explain difficult problems in a clear and understandable way.

We miss him terribly.

CONTENTS

LIST OF CONTRIBUTORS

John Brown DVM, PhD
Professor, Georgia Poultry Laboratory
Keith R Gooderham BVSc, MRCVS, DPMP
Poultry Veterinary Consultant
Mark A Goodwin DVM, MAM, PhD, Dipl. ACPV
Veterinary Pathologist and Associate Professor, Georgia
Poultry Laboratory
Nigel E Horrox BA, BVM&S, MRCVS
Poultry Veterinary Surgeon, Nigel Horrox Veterinary Group
Peter Hunton BSc, PhD
Consultant, Poultry Specialist, Ontario Egg Producers'
Marketing Board
Mark Pattison BVSc, MSc, PhD, MRCVS, DPMP
Head of Veterinary Services and Group Technical Manager,
Sun Valley Poultry Ltd.
Lucy M Rowland MS, MLS
Head, Science Collections and Branch Services, Georgia
Poultry Laboratory
D W B Sainsbury MA, PhD, MRCVS, F.I. Biol.
Lecturer in Animal Health, Department of Clinical
Veterinary Medicine, University of Cambridge
David Speight BSc, Dipl. Ag.
Consultant
J C Stuart BVSc, MRCVS, DPMP (deceased)

LIST OF COLOUR PLATES (Pages 128–9)

FOREWORD

Harold Temperton wrote in 1961, when Head of the National Institute of Poultry Husbandry, 'In the short space of forty years poultry keeping in Great Britain has attained the stature of a great specialised industry . . .'. This was true of many Western nations, but even so, the last 30 years has seen an equally dramatic development in the poultry industry of developed nations and, as importantly, a rapid development in scale and sophistication of poultry farming in the developing world. Eggs and poultry meat now form a major component of the animal protein in the diet of the population of the western world and in many of the developing nations. For example, world egg production has increased over two-fold and world poultry meat four and a half fold in the last 30 years.

Over this same period there have been dramatic developments in the prevention and control of many of the most devastating diseases of poultry. However, disease has, and will always have, a major potential for causing serious loss of poultry and compromising the efficiency of poultry production. A characteristic of many problems facing the veterinarian today are not traditional overt disease but diseases that reduce production. Although many of the major killers of poultry can now be controlled, they and many diseases that cause loss of production can only be prevented and controlled if attention is paid to all aspects of poultry husbandry. There are a number of textbooks on diseases and their causes. These provide the latest knowledge of each disease, its development, the causative agents and their properties together with approaches to their prevention and control. However, they focus quite intentionally on disease rather than health. This book recognizes that in the field most disease problems are multifactorial in cause and that the use of all the available components of that multifactorial cause to contribute to prevention and control is what is necessary, thus providing a positive approach to health. This approach is unique as far as textbooks are concerned.

The Editor, a renowned poultry practitioner, has assembled a distinguished group of experts who comprehensively cover all those aspects of poultry production that in some way can contribute to the health of the poultry flock. It is for these many reasons that this book will be welcomed and will, I am sure, find its way onto the bookshelves of all those connected with the poultry industry whether they are students, veterinarians, or managers.

Professor P M Biggs CBE, FRCVS, DSc, DVM, FRC Path.,
C Biol., F. I. Biol., FRS
Formerly Director, Houghton Poultry Research Station
November 1992

PREFACE & ACKNOWLEDGEMENTS

There are several standard textbooks which give good descriptions of all the known poultry diseases. It is not the purpose of this book to categorize these diseases with their causal organisms. It was felt there was a need for a text which looked at the overall concept of poultry health, to demonstrate the interrelationship between husbandry, medicine and nutrition in the prevention and treatment of disease. This book is therefore intended not only for poultry veterinarians but as a general veterinary text for agricultural and veterinary students, farmers and poultry production managers.

The modern poultry breeds, whether broiler or egg layer, achieve performance levels which would have been unheard of ten years ago, let alone 25 years ago when serious hybrid breeding really commenced. To achieve this genetic potential, all the important aspects of husbandry, nutrition and health must be working together in a strictly coordinated fashion.

The concept of preventive medicine in poultry is now more important than ever, because generally the occurrence of disease will limit the performance of the bird and prevent it from achieving its genetic potential. So often these days disease is not caused by a single agent (for which a clear-cut treatment or vaccine is available). More usually the disease is of multiple aetiology with several functions of management, nutrition and disease-producing agents involved. These problems, which may not be frank disease but rather suboptimum production, can often be difficult and time-consuming to solve. It is much better through a system of preventive medicine to avoid them happening in the first place.

Hence, to achieve maximum performance from poultry hybrids requires a close partnership between stockperson, nutritionist and veterinarian, and sympathetic management systems which allow this relationship to flourish. There is absolutely no question that good husbandry is as important with poultry as with any other species. The stockperson or flock manager ultimately holds the key to success assuming that he or she is provided with healthy birds, good feed, clean water, a suitable environment and good technical support when needed.

It is inevitable in a book of this kind that not all disease conditions can be mentioned. Also, the emphasis in different countries will vary according to the climate and geographical factors. It is more important for the reader to understand basic principles first, and then to use standard textbooks later for more detailed information as required.

The different sections of this book attempt to draw together some of the interrelating factors that contribute to this concept of a positive health status. The aim is to emphasize how important each aspect can be and to give the student an insight into how modern poultry husbandry is conducted.

Mark Pattison
May 1992

I would like to thank my wife Sue for all her support and advice in the production of this book. Thanks are due also to Mandy Harrold, Helen Hall and my daughter Emma for their cheerful and willing help with the typing of the manuscript, and to Norman Fincham for taking some of the photographs and to many other colleagues at Sun Valley Poultry who have helped in various ways.

We are indebted to the following for permission to reproduce copyright figures and tables:

The Cobb Breeding Company Ltd for Tables 6.2 & 6.3; the Controller of Her Majesty's Stationery Office for Table 4.10 (HMSO SI 1991 No. 2480); MS Technologies Ltd for Fig. 3.1; Ross Breeders Limited for Tables 6.1 & 6.4 (Ross Manual).

GENETICS AND BREEDING AS THEY AFFECT FLOCK HEALTH

PETER HUNTON, BSc, PhD

Introduction
Genetic resistance to disease
Eradication of vertically transmitted diseases
Breeder strategies for disease control
Conclusion

Introduction

The poultry industry can be represented as a pyramid (Figure 1.1). At the apex is a small group of primary breeders, with great-grandparent and grandparent stocks immediately below them. Most genetic selection takes place in the hands of the primary breeders, but some occurs among great-grandparent and grandparent flocks as well.

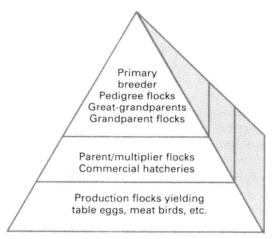

Figure 1.1 Hierarchical structure of the commercial poultry industry, showing genetic concentration of stock sources.

Below these sections, which represent relatively small numbers of birds, are the parent stocks, often called multiplier flocks, and below these are the commercial flocks which consist of meat birds or egg layers.

It is only in the period following World War II that the industry has evolved in this manner. Several factors combined to stimulate this development. One of the most important was the realization that the science of genetics could be harnessed to produce rapid genetic improvement in specialized strains of poultry developed for specific production purposes. Prior to this time, the industry had consisted of many relatively small hatcheries, drawing supplies of hatching eggs from their own or independent breeding flocks. Genetic quality was maintained by occasional purchases of stock from known superior breeders, plus a reliance on good stockmanship and the ability to distinguish healthy from unhealthy birds. Frequently, breeding flocks were not used to produce hatching eggs until their second laying season. This permitted natural selection for disease resistance and what the breeders of the time called 'vigour'. As the poultry industry became specialized into meat and egg sectors, the breeders responded by providing specialist types of bird for each sector. Individual breeders emerged who were demonstrably superior in particular types of stock: some bred egg production stocks, some broiler females, others broiler males, and quite separate companies established themselves in the breeding of turkeys.

A number of professional geneticists joined the poultry industry in the decade following World War II, and the number of primary breeders began to decline as those who failed to provide the competitive improvements, year by year, fell by the wayside.

Another factor which encouraged the development of a single purpose, primary breeding industry, was the adoption of modern methods for marketing and distribution of the products. Breeders with a superior product to sell developed franchise hatchery outlets and supported them with advertising, technical backup, and other marketing skills to increase market penetration.

Simultaneously, the development of international air transport made it possible for a breeder located anywhere in the world to achieve international distribution. It is entirely possible to transport chicks from a strategically located hatchery half-way around the world and place them within 24 hours, with very low mortality. Thus, grandparent and parent stocks could be distributed to remote customers, further increasing the market penetration on a world basis.

Besides its influence on the genetic characteristics of the world's poultry population, this structure has also had a profound influence on the incidence, prevention and spread of infectious diseases.

The number of primary breeders whose stocks make significant contributions to the world's poultry flocks has diminished rapidly. In 1990, three companies supplied most of the turkeys, six provided laying stock, and nine provided meat chickens for most of the world's industries. It will quickly become apparent that this situation renders commercial producers vulnerable to serious consequences relative to health, as well as production factors, should one of the major breeders, or several of them, suffer unexpected disease outbreaks or other problems. It also makes the commercial industry totally dependent upon the international breeders for maintaining their predicted rates of genetic progress. Failure to do this renders their customers extremely vulnerable to competition. This vulnerability is even more important in terms of the health of commercial generations. Diseases inadvertently transmitted with parents or grandparents, or susceptibility to unknown pathogens in remote countries can produce devastating results in the commercial poultry industry. The significance of industry structure with respect to flock health is not difficult to appreciate. Because many hundreds or thousands of commercial individuals are descended from each bird in the primary breeder flocks, it follows that the disease status, immune system, and genotype of the ancestor birds have potentially profound effects on the health of commercial flocks. The term 'biological multiplier effect' was coined some years ago for this phenomenon (Table 1.1).

Table 1.1 Biological multiplier effect. Approximate numbers of potential descendants from one pure line ancestor

Primary breeding flock	Generation			Commercial		
	Great-grandparent	Grand-parent	Parent	Birds	Tonnes	Eggs doz $\times$ 10^6
Meat type chickens						
Male line $\male$		100	1800	2×10^6	4000	
Female line $\female$	9	240	6000	780 000	1560	
Egg layers $\male$	–	480	400 000	300×10^6	–	6000
$\female$	–	40	3000	240 000	–	4.8

It is therefore entirely conceivable that any given layer or broiler flock, even a large one, could be traced back to literally a handful of birds at the primary breeder level.

We will examine, in the rest of this chapter, how this rigid industry structure affects the health of commercial poultry flocks. There are four separate pathways:

- genetic resistance to disease
- vertically transmitted (congenital) diseases

- parent immunocompetence
- control of horizontally transmitted diseases

Genetic resistance to disease

It is often tempting to attribute to genetics all abnormalities for which no other satisfactory explanation can be found. For example, the appearance in newly hatched chicks of crooked toes, crossed beaks or exencephaly is frequently attributed to genetics, because their hatchmates appear normal and no nutritional or infectious diseases are apparent. The difficulty in explaining these abnormalities on a genetic basis is that perhaps hundreds of siblings hatched from the same parents appear normal, and the parents themselves do not exhibit the abnormalities. The situation is made even more confusing by the fact that a few conditions, for example the 'star gazer', have a well-documented genetic basis, being due to recessive semi-lethals, inherited in a Mendelian ratio. While lethal genes are of interest to geneticists, they play very little part in commercial poultry production, having been eliminated from the primary breeding flocks early in their development. Reviews of lethal genes occurring in the major poultry species may be found in *Poultry Breeding and Genetics* (Crawford 1990). The lethal is mentioned only as an extreme example of genetic control of viability. Of much greater interest and concern is the genetic interaction with infectious disease organisms and also with environmental factors. Hutt (1958) provided some early examples of these which still stand. Gavora (1990) provides a discussion of much greater complexity with respect to genetic resistance to disease. In fact, in his introduction to a discussion of genetic variation in resistance to specific diseases, Gavora states: 'From early investigations up to the present time, genetic variation has been, almost without exception, found whenever adequately searched for.' The presence of genetic variation for resistance to disease carries with it the implication that (a) deliberate selection for improved resistance should provide positive results and (b) different strains may possess different levels of genetic resistance either as a result of chance or previous selection history. Although prior to domestication, poultry would have been expected to evolve in some kind of harmony with potential pathogens, the advent of artificial selection will have interfered with this to a considerable extent. Clearly, selection in the absence of pathogens, which most breeders strive to accomplish, provides a neutral environment as far as the development of genetic resistance to disease is concerned. However, there are various reasons for breeders' decisions in the area of breeding for disease resistance, and these will be dealt with later in this chapter.

Table 1.2 provides examples of genetic resistance to a variety of diseases in poultry.

Table 1.2 Examples of genetic resistance to specific infectious diseases and parasites

Disease	Reference
Pullorum disease (*Salmonella pullorum*)	Roberts and Card (1935) *Illinois Ag Exp Sta Bull* 419
Fowl typhoid (*Salmonella gallinarum*)	Hutt and Scholes (1941) *Poultry Science* 20: 342
Fowl typhoid in turkeys	Saif *et al.* (1984) *Avian Diseases* 28: 770
Turkey erysipelas	Saif *et al.* (1984) *Avian Diseases* 28: 770
Coccidiosis	Rosenberg *et al.* (1954) *Poultry Science* 33: 972
	Mathis *et al.* (1984) *Theoretical & Applied Genetics* 68: 385
Leucocytozoonosis (*Leucocytozoon caulleryi*)	Okada *et al.* (1988) *Proc. 18th World Poultry Congress, Nagoya*, p. 486
Nematode worms (*Acuaria lineata*)	Ackert *et al.* (1935) *Journal of Agricultural Research* 50: 607
(*A. galli*)	Buchwalder *et al.* (1977) *Monat Veterinärmed* 32: 898
Northern fowl mite (*Ornithoyssus sylviarum*)	Hall and Gross (1975) *Journal of Parasitology* 61: 1096 Eklund *et al.* (1980) *Archiv Geflügelk* 44: 195–9
Marek's disease	Hutt and Cole (1947) *Science* 106: 379
	Gavora 1990 (review) *Poultry Breeding and Genetics*, Elsevier
Lymphoid leukosis	Crittenden (1975) *Avian Diseases* 19: 281
Newcastle disease	Cole and Hutt (1961) *Avian Diseases* 5: 205
	Gordon *et al.* (1971) *Poultry Science* 50: 783
Avian encephalomyelitis	Hunton (1965) Unpublished
Infectious bronchitis and *E. coli*	Bumstead *et al.* (1989) *British Poultry Science* 30: 39

There are several other disease conditions for which no infectious cause has been found, but which appear to be under some degree of genetic control. These include pendulous crop in turkeys, perosis and other forms of leg weakness in broiler chickens and turkeys, and a variety of other diseases which will be considered later. However, while a genetic influence may exist, it is certainly not the only, and may not be the most important, factor in determining whether or not the disease appears. The same difficulty exists as with the abnormal day-old chicks, i.e. the temptation is to attribute the condition to genetics; but this ignores the fact that siblings may not exhibit the condition— the parents certainly did not.

Although broilers with generalized leg weakness may not exhibit clinical signs of disease, underlying infections may serve to aggravate the condition, or to cause it to become apparent when this would not have been the case in disease-free birds.

With infectious diseases, there are also many factors other than genetic resistance/susceptibility, a combination of which will determine whether or not individual birds exhibit signs of, or possibly die from, a specific disease. Among these factors, in addition to genetic resistance, are the following:

- presence or absence of pathogen
- concentration of pathogen
- maternal immunity
- immunocompetence of affected bird
- previous infection with same pathogen, leading to improved antibody status
- vaccination leading to improved antibody status
- genetic resistance to development of signs
- combination of some or all of the above, provoking recovery or progression of disease

Breeding companies are acutely aware of the potential for genetically determined disease resistance/susceptibility to influence the commercial success of their products. It would obviously be of great commercial advantage for a breeder to market a product with recognizable resistance to one or more specific diseases. However, the situation is much more complex than this statement implies. Because of the need to provide evidence of freedom from many diseases in sales, marketing and export documentation, breeders go to extreme lengths to minimize the presence of disease on their foundation stock farms. Extremely high levels of biosecurity are commonplace, to the extent that only a limited number of people have access to the farms. Feed and other necessary items taken onto the farm are carefully monitored, and all possible steps are taken to prevent disease entering the facilities. Only birds hatched from the breeder's own eggs will be placed on the foundation stock breeding farms. If birds are brought in from outside, they would normally be placed in quarantine. Thus the entire thrust of management is to provide freedom from disease, and to breed for maximum expression of economic traits. Under these circumstances, resistance or susceptibility to specific diseases will not be apparent, and may go completely unrecognized. In specific cases, breeding programmes were developed to circumvent these problems, and we will deal with some of these in the following sections.

Marek's disease

Marek's disease has been described as 'the most common of the lymphoproliferative diseases of chickens' (Calnek and Witter 1984). It is caused by a herpesvirus, is easily transmitted from bird to bird, and indeed the virus can be found in almost every flock of commercial birds in existence. Although the virus primarily attacks the nerves, causing paralysis, various other manifestations have been noted from time to time. Further complicating the literature on Marek's disease is the fact that it was only differentiated from lymphoid leukosis in the late 1960s. Prior to that, it was included in what was known as the 'leukosis complex'.

In the classical form, the disease attacks young birds from about five weeks of age onwards. Signs include various manifestations of paralysis of one or more limbs, and, in the case of acute outbreaks, high levels of mortality.

Several vaccines which provide good control of Marek's disease were developed and marketed in the early 1970s. However, prior to this, considerable evidence of genetic resistance to Marek's disease was apparent. Although in the early stages of their work, Hutt and Cole (Hutt 1958) did not distinguish between lymphoid leukosis and Marek's disease, they nevertheless developed strains exhibiting extremes of susceptibility and resistance. Hutt (1958) described the first 20 years of this experiment, and Cole and Hutt (1973) provided further evidence and were able to distinguish between resistance to the two diseases. Hutt and Cole developed two resistant lines (C and K) and one susceptible line (S) beginning in 1935. They did this by deliberately exposing young chickens to the environment of their parents. Selection criteria in these strains, in addition to resistance or susceptibility to leukosis, also included economic criteria such as egg production, egg size, etc.

This long-term experiment demonstrated clearly that genetic variation existed in the original lines for resistance to Marek's disease. When differential diagnosis became available, distinguishing Marek's disease from lymphoid leukosis, another experiment was initiated by Dr R. K. Cole, specifically aimed at demonstrating genetic resistance for Marek's disease. He used a broad-based population of White Leghorns, and deliberately exposed the growing birds by injecting them with a suspension of Marek's disease tumour cells. In only four generations (Cole 1972) the populations diverged so that in response to the same challenge, the resistant (N) line showed only 4.0% susceptibility, while the susceptible (P) line had a level of 91.5%. In the case of Cole's experiment, it was possible to breed from survivors of the artificial infection. Many commercial breeders adopted a variation of this system. Subpopulations of their main selection lines were exposed to the disease in isolated facilities, and then their sibs or parents were selected for breeding based on the incidence of tumours in the exposed population. There is no doubt that this procedure enabled several breeders to improve the genetic resistance of their stocks to Marek's disease. The practice was concentrated in the egg-laying stocks, since these were the ones which appeared to suffer the greatest loss from field exposure to the disease. However, the cost of this research was extremely high, and when vaccines were marketed in the early 1970s, most commercial breeders abandoned the concept. However, while vaccines provided excellent protection, evidence was later published (Gavora and Spencer 1979) indicating clearly that even among vaccinated birds, those with higher genetic resistance showed lower mortality in response to challenge than did birds with genetic susceptibiity.

The rapid progress made by Cole in his development of the N and P lines suggested the possibility of a single gene with a disproportionately large effect on resistance to Marek's disease. Briles *et al.* (1977) reported a gene at the *B*-locus of the major histocompatibility complex (MHC) which appeared to confer resistance to Marek's disease. This gene, identified as B^{21}, was subsequently found to be homozygous in Cole's N line, but absent from Hutt and Cole's C and K lines. Gavora (1990) identified a number of lines in which B^{21} and, to a smaller extent, B^2 conferred resistance to Marek's disease or in which frequencies of these alleles increased as a consequence of selection for resistance.

There are many different strains of Marek's disease virus (Calnek and Witter 1984). These show considerable variation in virulence and pathogenicity. Vaccines have been prepared from mild, non-pathogenic strains, from virulent strains which have been attenuated in the laboratory, or from the related herpes virus of turkeys. The vaccines appear to work by preventing development of signs of Marek's disease.

However, they apparently do not prevent infection of the hosts with the Marek's disease virus: virus can be recovered from almost any commercial chickens tested. Similarly, the mode of action of the resistant genes is not clear either. Thus the possibility remains that a 'new' virus might develop which could circumvent the effects of vaccines and/or those of genetic resistance. Overcoming the effects of vaccines would initially restore responsibility for preventing the disease to the breeders. Genetic resistance would again become the first line of defence, provided that the 'new' virus did not also overcome this protection.

Lymphoid leukosis

Crittenden (1975) described two levels of genetic resistance to lymphoid leukosis (LL). The first is cellular resistance to infection by the virus, and the second is the resistance of infected birds to the development of tumours. There are at least four subgroups of LL virus, and cellular resistance to each of them is controlled by a single allele. In the case of subgroups A, B and C, the alleles for susceptibility are dominant over those for resistance. This means that an individual classified as resistant possesses the recessive, resistant allele at both loci, and would pass this gene to all its progeny. Relatively simple laboratory tests using tissue culture or chick embryos are available to identify these alleles. Thus the necessity for using growing birds infected with the virus for subsequent autopsy is avoided. However, while the existence of these genes provides an opportunity for breeders to incorporate resistance to the common subgroups of LL (A and B), their distribution in different populations has prevented large-scale application. Most White Leghorn strains appear to be homozygous for the susceptible alleles. Thus breeders are faced with introducing the allele from other populations, or developing alternative strategies to produce resistant products. On the other hand, many of the strains used in the production of brown egg and meat stocks of chickens carry the alleles for resistance, and some progress has been made in incorporating these into commercial products. There is some circumstantial evidence to indicate that such incorporation does indeed provide protection from LL mortality.

Notwithstanding the usefulness of resistant alleles in controlling the disease, the breeding system is still exposed to the risk that new subgroups of the virus might enter populations, and unless resistant alleles were discovered, these could provide new sources of disease.

Furthermore, while the diseases are caused by exogenous viruses, endogenous viruses are carried by almost all individuals which complicates the process of identifying exogenous viruses and their antigens.

The second aspect of genetic resistance refers to the ability of infected birds to resist tumour development. Gyles *et al.* (1981) reported a series of experiments to develop genetically selected lines in which tumours would regress. Modest heritabilities were noted for days-to-regression of a tumour induced by inoculation of Rous sarcoma virus.

Part of the genetic contribution to leukosis resistance at this level is also related to B-alleles at the MHC. While not nearly as consistent as the apparent resistance to Marek's disease conferred by the B^{21} allele, B^2 has been observed to enhance resistance to various challenges with Rous sarcoma and LL viruses (Bacon 1987). Bacon has also demonstrated that different B haplotypes differ in the rate at which they shed LL virus.

The presence of LL virus in an individual or a population is not necessarily an indication of potential mortality. Indeed, mortality may not be the most important source of economic loss from LL. Gavora *et al.* (1980) have shown that in several White Leghorn populations, LL virus shedders have delayed maturity and lower egg production than non-shedders from the same populations. And although very few birds in these flocks died from LL, mortality from other causes was more than double among the LL virus shedders compared with the non-shedders.

Because lymphoid leukosis is transmitted both vertically and horizontally, breeders have attempted to eradicate the virus from their foundation breeding stocks, and thus have placed themselves in a position to distribute stock free of the disease. Strict biosecurity and hygiene can minimize the risk of horizontal transmission to such flocks, and in this way the commercial products may be protected from the disease.

Eradication of vertically transmitted diseases

Salmonella species

The first disease of economic importance to be addressed through eradication procedures was pullorum disease, caused by *Salmonella pullorum*. This salmonella is unique in that it is pathogenic only to chickens, to a lesser degree for the turkey, and of very little importance in other species. However, young infected chickens show high levels of mortality, following acute signs of diarrhoea. The salmonella organisms are transmitted from carrier hens, which may not show signs, to hatching eggs, and thence into the newly hatched chicks. Evidence of infection may be observed in the hatchery, but usually it is not seen until a few days after hatching. Thus large numbers of infected chicks could be distributed from a single hatchery, and this was the main method of spread of the disease in the early days of the poultry industry. Chicks receiving the infection from their dams would also horizontally infect hatch-mates, leading to high levels of morbidity and mortality. Mortality varies from trivial up to 100%, usually during the second week after hatching.

Birds which recover from an outbreak remain carriers, and may potentially pass the infection to their own offspring.

Fortunately for the poultry industry, recovered birds, besides carrying the bacterium, also develop recognizable antibodies. Commercial antigens have subsequently been developed which can be used to detect antibodies in whole blood using the rapid plate test or tube agglutination tests.

Because of the widespread nature of pullorum disease, and because it was clearly spread from hatcheries, many national, government sponsored control programmes were established to eradicate the condition. Examples are the Poultry Stock Improvement Plan (later the Poultry Health Scheme) in the UK and the National Poultry Improvement Program in the USA. These programmes developed protocols for the testing and certification of all parent stocks used to supply eggs to commercial hatcheries. Breeding flocks are blood-tested before hatching eggs are allowed to be drawn by the hatcheries. Reactor birds are identified and either retested or immediately withdrawn from the flock, which is then usually retested after a specified time interval. As a result of this, many countries have essentially eradicated *Salmonella pullorum* from their commercial layer, broiler and turkey industries.

At the same time as pullorum disease was being eradicated, another similar, but quite distinct disease, fowl typhoid, was also brought under control. Fowl typhoid is caused by the bacterium *Salmonella gallinarum*, which is detected by the same antigen used to detect *S. pullorum*.

Avian arizonosis is a significant economic problem in the turkey industry in the USA. Classification of the organism in the genus *Salmonella* has been proposed, although there are some minor variations in its characteristics from those normally associated with *Salmonella* spp. However, elimination of the organism from breeding flocks, by means of serological testing of parents and grandparents, has been successful in many instances in reducing the spread of Arizona infections. Most turkey breeding stocks sold today are free of infection.

Mycoplasma infections

Mycoplasma galliseticum

The success of eradication programmes for the various *Salmonella* species provided a model for dealing with mycoplasma infections. These began to emerge as serious problems in the broiler industry during the 1960s. *M. gallisepticum* was first associated with chronic respiratory disease in broilers. It was later found to impair reproductive performance in various ways in both meat-type breeders and egg-laying hens, and to be responsible for infectious sinusitis in turkeys. These diseases are frequently aggravated by other subclinical bacterial infections, and tend to be exaggerated under modern commercial management conditions, involving high density housing. While the impact of the diseases can be significantly reduced by attention to hygiene and management procedures, the fact remains that eradication of the organism is an achievable goal. Thus breeders have attempted to remove the organism from foundation and grandparent stocks. *M. gallisepticum* tends to spread rapidly from bird to bird, and therefore the identification and removal of carriers as a method of eradication proved to be impossible. Various antibiotics are effective in reducing *M. gallisepticum* infections. These may be applied at various levels. Medication of breeders will reduce the rate of egg transmission to low levels, but will not generally eradicate it. Pre-incubation immersion of warmed hatching eggs in cooler antibiotic solutions is another possibility, as is the inoculation of the fertile incubating eggs with antibiotic solution. Unfortunately, all these methods suffer the disadvantage that while the organism may, in fact, be eliminated, the antibodies are not, and it is therefore difficult to distinguish between infected and uninfected individuals.

Another useful technique in the eradication programme has been the high-temperature treatment of hatching eggs. *M. gallisepticum* (and *M. synovie*) have been found to be inactivated at temperatures of more than 46 °C. Hatching eggs heated to achieve this temperature internally suffer declines in hatchability, but in many cases yield progeny which do not carry the *Mycoplasma* species. Through a combination of these methods, *M. gallisepticum* has been largely eradicated from layer, broiler and turkey stocks. Freedom from the organism is verified by serology. Serum plate tests, haemagglutination inhibition (HI) tests and enzyme-linked immunosorbent assay (ELISA) have all been used in the detection of *M. gallisepticum.*

Mycoplasma synoviae

M. synoviae is another egg-transmitted infection prevalent in chickens and turkeys. Although the disease is easily spread by horizontal means, the initial egg transmission makes it another disease which can best be controlled by eradication at the primary breeder level. The methods of detection and eradication are very similar to those used for *M. gallisepticum.* Most chickens and turkeys now available from breeders are free of *M. synoviae.*

Mycoplasma meleagridis *infection*

M. meleagridis is a specific pathogen of turkeys, causing a respiratory disease similar to *M. gallisepticum.* Also it is thought that the hatchability of infected eggs is reduced. In addition to passage through the eggs, *M. meleagridis* may also be transmitted in semen. Control at the primary breeder level has been accomplished by culturing swabs from the reproductive tract of both sexes to detect carriers, and eliminating them. The treatment of eggs with antibiotics and the rearing of *M. meleagridis* negative stock in isolation have combined to eradicate the organism from most primary breeder stocks.

Lymphoid leukosis eradication

Since many White Leghorn lines appear not to carry the genes coding for resistance to the LL viruses, the breeders have tended to take the approach of eradication. Various methods for detecting the LL infection, or antigens provoked by these viruses, have been used. Some of these efforts have been made more difficult by the existence of the endogenous virus genes present in most stocks. Because these genes are very similar in antigenicity to the exogenous LL viruses, some tests cannot distinguish between them, and the populations appear to continue to be LL positive, even when most of the exogenous viruses have been eradicated. The endogenous genes appear to vary in frequency, mainly in response to selection for high productivity, since they appear to be mildly disadvantageous to reproductive success. A discussion of these inter-relationships has been provided by Kuhnlein *et al.* (1989) and the subject is reviewed by Gavora (1990).

Breeder strategies for disease control

Both the development of genetic resistance to disease, and the eradication of specific pathogens from foundation stocks, commit breeders to large expenditures and to the use of resources which might provide greater economic progress if utilized in other applications. In many cases the successful control of diseases by drug therapy and/or vaccination has encouraged breeders to abandon efforts to control them by eradicating pathogens or selecting for genetic resistance. For example, the very high cost of exposing subpopulations to direct challenge with Marek's disease meant that this practice was quickly abandoned with the introduction of successful vaccines. The emergence of other methods of detecting genetic resistance to Marek's disease, for example selection for specific alleles of the major histocompatibility complex, which could be accomplished at least at the research level, without exposing individuals to the disease, provoked a renewal of interest in genetic resistance to Marek's disease.

Bacon's (1987) review of the influence of the MHC on disease resistance and productivity traits indicates several possible methods by which breeders might develop new or improved stocks.

The technical capability of identifying B-alleles for Marek's resistance might be further extended to those influencing other diseases such as lymphoid leukosis. Once a breeder has acquired the resources for work in this area, other applications become increasingly attractive. Rapid investigation and application of published research are possible when these affect economically important factors of concern to breeders and their customers.

While this discussion might lead to the belief that breeders' strategies in this area are largely opportunistic, such is not the case. A combination of intense competition, plus rigorous international phytosanitary regulations, leaves little room for choice in many cases. For many years breeding stocks have had to be free of S. pullorum, S. gallinarum and the important Mycoplasma species. Increasing concern with food safety led some countries to broaden the spectrum of reportable Salmonella serotypes to include those responsible for human illnesses in addition to poultry pathogens. Under these circumstances, breeders test for and attempt to control a wide range of salmonellae and thus offer for sale breeding stocks free of any detectable infection with this species. Because of the chance of recontamination, this Salmonella-free status may not be guaranteed but it is likely to be a fact in the majority of shipments.

With cheap and effective vaccines available for many virus diseases, there is little incentive for breeders to become involved in complex selection programmes for genetic resistance to them. The exceptions to this generalization are Marek's disease and possibly lymphoid leukosis. There is no vaccine available for leukosis, and it has been clearly shown that stocks genetically resistant to Marek's disease do better, even when vaccinated, than susceptible stocks when exposed to field challenges.

Accepting this, however, breeders are extremely concerned to provide for sale stocks with a high level of immunocompetence, so that they will respond effectively to vaccination. While genetic factors affecting immunocompetence are elusive, much can be achieved by ensuring control of immunosuppressive conditions such as infectious bursal disease.

For diseases which are controlled largely by drug therapy, different priorities apply which may impact on breeders. Probably the best example in this class is coccidiosis. Historically, coccidiosis has been controlled by preventive drug therapy. A series of chemicals, to which coccidia eventually become resistant, have been developed. Even though evidence of genetic resistance to coccidiosis exists, chemotherapy has remained the control method of choice.

Immunocompetence: the contribution of the breeder

Because many of the diseases associated with intensive poultry production are controlled by vaccination, it is important to ensure that successive generations of birds are able to respond to the antigens provided and develop immunity. Several known factors may compromise this ability, and some of them are under the control of breeders and multipliers.

Maternal immunity affords protection to early disease challenges, but it may also interfere with response to early vaccinations. Experience has shown that maternal immunity is measurable and predictable and, in combination with the appropriate choice of vaccines, can be effectively utilized and accounted for.

Of greater importance are diseases which suppress the immune system, rendering vaccinations partly or wholly ineffective. The best known of these is infectious bursal disease (IBD) or Gumboro disease (named after Gumboro, Delaware, where it was first observed). Breeders and hatcheries are involved with IBD because the status of any flock with respect to the disease determines the status of its progeny. When the disease was originally discovered among commercial broilers, it became evident that some breeders' premises were not contaminated with the causal virus, presumably as a result of biosecurity efforts. However, since they lacked maternal immunity, breeding stock originating from such premises were extremly susceptible to field exposure. If they survived without exposure, their commercial progeny were equally susceptible and, because of the widespread nature of the disease, almost certain to be exposed.

Thus, at every generation, IBD status must be assessed and appropriate vaccination programmes developed so that progeny have the highest possible level of immunocompetence.

Marek's disease is also involved in immunosuppression, although its primary signs of paralysis and mortality are much more obvious. Because almost all commercial chickens are vaccinated for Marek's disease, the immunosuppressive effects are not so well defined or recognized.

Non-specific diseases with genetic implications

Breeders have made major changes in the genotypes of commercial chickens since serious selection programmes became part of poultry breeding midway through the 20th century. This is nowhere more visible than in the case of meat chickens and turkeys, but it is also evident, though perhaps less spectacular, in both white and brown egg-laying stocks. Illustrations of the change in performance of chicken broilers and egg layers are given in Table 1.3. These

Table 1.3 Changes in broiler and layer performance, 1950–1988

Year	Broilers[1] (Days to reach 1820 g liveweight)	Layers[2] (Eggs/hen/year)
1950	84	120
1960	70	157
1970	59	216
1980	51	242
1988	44	260

[1] Adapted from Gyles (1989).
[2] Adapted from Hartmann (1990).

changes are the result of genetic, nutrition, and health improvements, along with major changes in management practices. They have led to the emergence of a number of conditions, which might be broadly classified as diseases, which seem to be strictly related to the high level of performance exhibited by the modern chicken and turkey stocks. These conditions may be aggravated by environmental factors or by otherwise non-pathogenic disease organisms. The following are examples:

- various forms of leg weakness in meat chickens and turkeys
- ascites in meat chickens
- deep pectoral myopathy in turkeys (and possibly chickens)
- excessive decline in eggshell quality with age in layers
- caged layer fatigue

Leg weakness in broilers and turkeys

The emergence of leg weaknesses in meat birds as a significant economic problem became evident in the 1970s and 1980s. Confusion arose because of problems of nomenclature: twisted legs, perosis, leg weakness, dyschondroplasia and many other terms have been used in industry. Julian (1990a) has proposed a system of standard terminology which will be used here. The objective of this discussion is not so much to describe the conditions, as to indicate the part played by genetics in their appearance. According to Julian (1990a), up to 60% of the lameness observed among broiler chickens and 30–40% of that in turkeys results from a condition described as angular bone deformity, twisted legs or valgus-varus deformity. Tibial dyschondroplasia (TD) and spondylolisthesis among broiler chickens are the other major contributors.

Because most of the conditions including the term 'leg weakness' have been ill defined, it is not surprising that solutions to the various problems have not always been obvious. And the implication of genetics is, at best, tenuous. Difficulties arise because the incidence of the conditions is sporadic, and often seems to be influenced by non-genetic factors such as nutrition, housing density, immune status of birds, toxins and the presence or absence of other diseases. Furthermore, the conditions are seldom seen among pure line stocks belonging to primary breeder flocks, among which selection against such traits might be practised. In fact, for many years breeders have gone to considerable lengths to improve leg strength in their pure lines, particularly among ancestors of male parent stocks. Strategies include careful observation of the birds' anatomy during early selections, and subsequent culling of any birds exhibiting abnormalities of gait or posture.

However, several studies, of which Wong-Valle et al. (1990) is the most recent, have indicated that the incidence of TD, which can be fairly well defined, can be modified by selection. Similar evidence exists that shank width may be influenced by selection. In the experiment of Wong-Valle et al. (1990), it was shown that a significant difference in the incidence of TD could be achieved in only two generations of selection in opposite directions. They and others have observed no differences in body weight between high and low incidence lines. The implication here is that in circumstances of intense selection for body-weight increase, there should be no natural selection favouring the emergence of TD as a problem.

Yet field evidence suggests that this and other leg problems are more frequently observed in rapidly growing flocks and seem, if anything, to be increasing in incidence. The explanation must involve a degree of genetic susceptibility, but must also include a number of nutritional, environmental and pathological factors which vary between flocks, and even between birds within flocks. It is the combination of these factors, along with genetics, which determines the presence or absence of any particular condition.

Ascites in meat chickens

Although ascites is generally defined as an excessive accumulation of serous fluid in the abdominal cavity, the condition referred to here specifically relates only to meat chickens, and is the result of right heart failure. This condition, like some of the leg problems described previously, is not genetic in the sense of being the result of lethal genes. Rather, it is a complex condition, the incidence of which seems to have increased substantially among the rapidly growing broiler and roaster chickens that result from prolonged selection for meat characteristics and rapid growth rate.

Julian (1990b) has provided an excellent description of the condition as it appears in modern broiler flocks. He has also provided details concerning various factors which contribute to pulmonary hypertension and right heart failure. Among these are predisposing environmental factors which may combine to increase the incidence of ascites or, if controlled, may limit or eliminate it. They include:

- high altitude, with resulting hypoxia
- low temperature, leading to increased oxygen requirement
- aspergillosis, impairing lung function
- reduced oxygen-carrying capacity of the blood, as a result of elevated carbon monoxide levels

In fact, ascites has always been something of a problem at high altitudes. It is only during the latter part of the 20th century that it has emerged as a problem among broilers grown at low altitudes.

The most important factor associated with a high incidence of ascites appears to be the increased oxygen demand created by rapid growth. Increasing growth rates are a fact of life in chicken production. Julian (1990c) has stated: 'Selection for rapid growth and muscle mass on a small skeleton has produced a chicken that has insufficient capacity for blood-flow to supply its body's oxygen requirement during periods of rapid growth.' He also asks: 'If genetics has produced the problem, can it also provide a solution that does not involve slowing growth?'

Testing of pedigreed stocks in low temperatures and/or high altitude conditions would quickly reveal evidence of genetic variation, but sustained selection for this type of trait would not only be very expensive but would inevitably divert selection effort away from other characteristics. However, with the background of the disease so well defined, and with no pathogen directly involved, the call for a genetic solution to the problem may have considerable merit.

Caged layer fatigue and impaired shell quality

Caged layer fatigue, more commonly known as osteoporosis, is a condition observed occasionally in laying flocks producing at high rates of lay. The condition is characterized by extreme fragility, and sometimes fractures of some of the cortical bones, particularly those of the ribs and limbs. Birds suffering from this condition suffer partial or complete paralysis, and usually die from dehydration if they cannot reach a water source. Impaired shell quality is usually a function of age or other factors. Although these two conditions are considered together here, they seldom occur together in commercial flocks.

The reason for considering these two conditions together arises from the fact that both relate to the metabolism, utilization and distribution of calcium. In the modern laying hen, the need for and utilization of calcium is extremely critical. A hen which lays 300 eggs in a year in fact lays down 600 g of calcium (1.6 kg of calcium carbonate) in a 12-month period. On a daily basis, when an eggshell is produced, 2.0 g of calcium must be laid down through the agency of a blood supply which contains no more than 25 mg at any given time. Thus producing a shell in 18 hours requires the hen to lay down 110 mg/hour, or a total turnover of blood calcium every 12 minutes.

The source of calcium for eggshell formation consists of a combination of dietary calcium and medullary bone reserves. Dietary calcium is absorbed in the alimentary tract and transferred via the bloodstream to either the shell gland directly or to temporary storage in medullary bone. Medullary bone reserves are utilized during eggshell formation.

In the case of caged layer fatigue, some poorly understood factors result in the upsetting of the calcium balance, depletion of medullary bone reserves and also calcium from some of the cortical bones. Birds showing signs of osteoporosis are usually in full production and frequently have a partially shelled egg in the shell gland post-mortem.

As birds age, shell quality tends to deteriorate to varying extents. Egg size increases with age, and with this the amount of calcium required to produce a good quality shell increases as well. However, although the requirement for calcium on the day that an egg is laid increases with egg-size increase, this is partly compensated by increased time between ovipositions and more frequent interruptions to the sequence of eggs providing greater opportunities for the repletion of calcium reserves.

Why should these conditions form part of a discussion of the effects of genetics and breeding? Modern layers result from many generations of selection for such traits as early sexual maturity, increasing rate of lay, and reduced body weight. Selection has also been aimed at improving shell quality, using various criteria, mainly physical or mechanical measurements of the shell. No direct assessments of 'calcium efficiency' have been possible, and therefore the influence which selection has had on calcium metabolism is, if present, only indirect.

It is hypothesized that geneticists have inadvertently moved high-producing laying flocks closer to some threshold, beyond which calcium metabolism can no longer serve the competing demands of shell production and bone maintenance. There is good evidence of significant genetic variation in many measures of eggshell quality, and some indication that strains vary in their expression of osteoporosis.

The response of hens is clearly influenced by many environmental factors. Among these are calcium source, calcium particle size, the level of other elements, particularly phosphorus in the diet, and the level and form of vitamins particularly vitamin D. In addition, shell quality deterioration seems to be influenced by a number of infectious diseases, particularly viruses which affect both the respiratory and reproductive tracts. While not directly related to shell quality, it is interesting to note that Spackman (1985) reported virtually no decline in albumen quality of specific pathogen-free hens, while normal commercial flocks showed significant reductions. It is possible that this might also be the case for shell quality deterioration.

Deep pectoral myopathy

This condition was first described in turkeys, but has also been noted occasionally in meat-type chickens (Grunder et al. 1984). The disease was originally discovered in Oregon, hence it was referred to as 'Oregon disease' and has also been known as green muscle disease. For a concise description and a review of the causative factors, pathology and a discussion of the disease and its ramifications, the reader is referred to Siller (1985).

Spontaneous occurrence of the disease is seen mainly in spent breeder turkey hens, and its incidence is thought to be due to the birds' struggling and wing beating associated with catching for artificial insemination. Although it is not of economic significance among growing turkeys or broilers, the disease is sufficiently serious to be of concern, particularly in view of the potential for increasing incidence, as further increases in growth rate and body size result from genetic, nutritional and environmental developments.

Evidence of genetic variation in the incidence of deep pectoral myopathy was presented early in its history by Harper et al. (1975) based on their studies at Oregon State University. In his review, Siller (1985) concludes that 'it is a condition coincidental with the production of large breasted turkeys and broilers, and is therefore a penalty of successful selection!'

Direct evidence that susceptibility to the condition would respond to selection is lacking. However, the fact that the disease occurs only in populations with a long selection history for increased breast musculature suggests a genetic component. Whether or not breeders will ultimately include selection for this trait in their programme may depend upon a number of factors, including field incidence, the emergence of other preventive measures or the discovery of a sensitive indicator of susceptibility.

Conclusion

The structure of the poultry meat and egg production industries provides both challenges and opportunities in the area of poultry health.

The challenges include breeding programmes tending to produce genetically uniform populations, selected in environments where infectious diseases are eliminated as far as possible. This process involves risks. It is possible that the progeny of these populations, when multiplied in commercial industry, might prove susceptible to diseases already present in the field. Or new strains of disease might emerge to which no natural resistance is present in breeders' stocks. Diminishing numbers of breeders, and the limited horizons within which competition compels them to work, tend to amplify this risk. Furthermore, because breeders all aim at very similar markets, it follows that real genetic differences between competing stocks may be very small indeed. Such differences as do exist may not relate to disease resistance, although there is some evidence that variation between different stocks, in susceptibility to Marek's disease, was observed prior to the introduction of vaccines. However, the very nature of the industry forces breeders to undertake rigorous field testing of new products before introducing them on a large scale. This helps ensure that newly developed stocks will be capable of competitive performance in, and survival under, commercial conditions of disease exposure.

A second challenge is the existence of very high-density populations of commercial poultry. Such circumstances provide an ideal medium for multiplication and spread of all kinds of microorganisms including pathogens. While not originally a genetic or breeding problem, growers have suggested a need for general disease resistance at the genetic level. While some research has been undertaken in this area, there has been little progress in practical terms. Some evidence exists that genotypes resistant to bacterial infection may be more susceptible to viruses, and *vice versa*. Until more detailed knowledge of these genetic systems becomes available, breeders must continue to rely on their non-genetic strategies, i.e. understanding the immune system and optimizing its competence by various means.

The possibility of a devastating new disease is always a potential threat to the poultry industry. The example most quoted is that of corn blight, which affected huge areas of the US corn (maize) crop in the 1970s. Few, if any, commercial varieties had genetic resistance, and no other methods of control were available. The history of the poultry industry contains examples of major diseases, which have been contained using drug therapy or prophylaxis, and preventive vaccination. There is no example of the sole use of genetic replacement, although in the case of Marek's disease, referred to above, this approach might have achieved more prominence had not an effective vaccine been introduced. The extent of disruption which the industry might experience, as a result of a new disease with no solution other than the introduction of new genotypes, is almost impossible to calculate. Assuming that resistant genotypes existed among breeders' stocks, a minimum of three to five years would be necessary for multiplication and distribution.

However, the previous discussion is a worst-case scenario. There is another aspect which clearly indicates that the industry structure provides a major advantage, and this is the ability to disseminate newly developed genotypes and disease-controlled stocks quickly and effectively. This applies equally to production traits and disease resistance factors. The virtual eradication of $S.$ $pullorum$ from commercial poultry is a case in point. Eradication of $M.$ $gallisepticum$ from the broiler industry is another example. However, the same cannot be said of the egg industry in the USA, which either through choice or indifference continued to tolerate the negative effects of $M.$ $gallisepticum$. The point here is that whether or not the disease was eradicated, breeders, by supplying grandparent and/or parent stock free of the infection, provided the opportunity for commercial generations to retain that status. Without the initiative of the breeding sector, the choice of eradication would not be available.

Another benefit conferred by the poultry industry's unique structure is the method whereby industrial needs are translated into genetic and breeding strategies. Because breeders' business is international in scope they are aware of the world-wide spectrum of disease conditions, as well as the changing requirements for other commercial traits. The recognition of the problem created by Marek's disease and the potential for applying newly published genetic research provided an excellent example of this in the late 1960s. Before Cole's work (Cole 1972) was formally published, several breeders had established facilities for applying it to their own populations and incorporating the genetic advances in the stock which they sold. Similarly, breeders' response to the discovery of IBD (Gumboro) and the need to develop and exploit parental immunity, using vaccines, enabled the industry to limit the damage resulting from this disease.

Finally the concentration of breeding and genetic development into relatively few hands, while carrying certain risks, also places responsibility with organizations possessing the resources necessary for maintaining continuity and product quality. In the evolution of the breeding industry some businesses failed, not because of inferior stock but through lack of the finance necessary to further develop and distribute the products. Breeders supplying the industry in the late 20th century tend to be associated with large, well-financed, multinational corporations. These organizations are able to maintain the costly infrastructure necessary for ongoing research and development. They are also able to provide marketing and support services as necessary in distributing improved stocks to the commercial industry.

The breeding and multiplication sectors of the poultry industry have made significant contributions to poultry health. Their status in the late 20th century provides a foundation from which continuing and new initiatives may be expected to grow.

Further Reading

Crawford R D (ed) (1990) *Poultry breeding and genetics*. Elsevier, Amsterdam, New York.

Hofstad M S, Barns H J, Calnek B W, Reid W M, Yoder H W Jr. (eds) (1991) *Diseases of poultry*. Iowa State College Press, Ames, Iowa.

Hutt F B (1949) *Genetics of the fowl*. McGraw-Hill, New York.

Hutt F B (1958) *Genetic resistance to disease in domestic animals*. Comstock Publishing Associates, Ithca, New York.

Jordan F T W (ed) (1990) *Poultry diseases* 3rd ed. Baillière Tindall, London.

2 POULTRY ENVIRONMENT, HOUSING AND HYGIENE
D. W. B. SAINSBURY, MA, PhD, MRCVS, F.I. Biol.

Introduction

The importance of ensuring the best possible design and quality of housing as a vital aid to the good production, welfare and health of poultry can hardly be exaggerated. Under this general heading many factors must be considered and are dealt with in this chapter, including:

1. The planning and siting of the unit.
2. Construction of the buildings.
3. The microclimate within the housing.
4. Ventilation, air movement and its control.
5. Lighting.
6. Hygiene and disinfection.
7. Overall management and choice of systems.
8. Welfare and alternative systems.

It needs to be emphasized that the advice of the veterinarian is vital at every stage and is especially important during the early planning of the unit when factors such as the size and siting of the enterprise are under consideration. Regrettably it is still exceptional for this to be done and many poultry farms are so badly conceived that they are destined either to function inefficiently or to become a total failure. It would not be difficult to make a list of many such enterprises in a large number of countries. The difficulty is to persuade the controlling business, commercial and financial interests of the importance of the veterinarian's input. It is hoped that the details set out in this chapter will help in correcting this omission.

Planning and siting of the unit

The siting of the poultry unit is an important factor to consider whatever type of housing is being erected. A first consideration is to place it as far away as possible from other poultry sites, or other potential sites. Many poultry pathogens can be windborne on particles of dust for long distances—evidence of 70 km at least has been given for the spread of pathogens from large intensive conglomerates. The site itself should be open, well drained, with a southerly aspect. A moderate slope will also help with drainage. On especially exposed sites attention should be given to the use of either existing or new trees as windbreaks. Special care must be taken with ventilation both on exposed sites where good baffling devices will be needed to reduce adventitious air flow and on sheltered sites where mechanical ventilation is almost invariably necessary. The positioning of the buildings on a site will depend to a great extent on the need to reduce movement to a minimum and to allow for easy handling of equipment, food and birds. Adequate roads and turning space, tailored to the size of vehicles to be used on the site, must be installed. Every care has to be taken, however, to ensure that attention to ease of movement does not result in the buildings being too close together, or the risk of disease transfer is greatly increased and good free ventilation is impaired. A sound principle with naturally ventilated houses is to allow a distance between buildings at least equal to the width of each building. Every site should have no other livestock on it or immediately adjoining it.

Site security

The poultry industries of the world are increasingly afflicted by near overwhelming virus infections that are spread by every imaginable route. The airborne route has already been mentioned. Not very much can be done about this except by attempting to locate sites as far apart as possible and by limiting their size (see later in this chapter). In addition every site needs to have special measures of security to prevent the entry of disease by mechanical means—from people, vehicles, livestock and equipment. A high and complete fence around the site with a locked gate is essential. Vehicles should go through a disinfectant dip and in emergency periods when virulent disease is near at hand, through a disinfectant spray. Ideally, and by no means an impractical proposition, feed lorries should deliver from outside the site by mechanically conveying or blowing feed into the bins within the site. Just inside the gateway there should be a 'hygiene station'—a building containing a changing room, toilets, showers, protective clothing and boots, and no access to the site should be possible without passing through this.

Site size

It is impossible to give exact advice as to what constitutes either the optimal or the maximum size of a poultry unit. Much depends on the standard of management; if this is very high it can handle large numbers of birds kept together. From personal observation with broiler poultry, units of up to 100 000 birds on one site can be satisfactory; above this the unit tends to become more tense but up to 200 000 on a site can work reasonably well. It would not be normal to advise more than this, but there are certainly some good units in the region of 300 000 birds. For commercial egg layers a size of up to 70 000 is satisfactory whilst for breeders up to 20 000 is a reasonably satisfactory maximum number.

It is well to bear in mind the overall evidence that the larger the site the poorer the biological results. A summary of investigations over many years gives examples of results with broilers. Best performance is on sites of about $600\,m^2$—a modest size, since that would take only about 12 000 birds. And for every doubling of the size above this, average weight decreased by 0.09 kg. Thus if birds attained 2 kg in a 12 000 bird unit, a 120 000 unit would give a weight of about 1.7 kg. Such a diminution of weight is usually accompanied by poorer food conversion efficiency and higher morbidity.

Husbandry, unit size and efficiency

It is one of the encouraging elements in poultry husbandry that, in spite of mass production methods and reliance on automation, birds are still highly responsive to the effects of management. No more and no less than other farm livestock, birds with the same apparent housing, nutrition and facilities, and of the same genetic material are still capable of giving *vastly* different results depending on the care taken with management. It is significant that usually the farms which head the tables of productivity are the smaller units in the personal charge of the owner. These are more efficient on several grounds as a way of producing *any* poultry products.

If productivity is better and food conversion improved, then clearly the world's resources are being used most economically. Thus the very large unit may seem profitable as a purely financial exercise because of the very large numbers of stock, but as a means of utilizing the world's limited resources this may not be so at all and if productivity, food conversion and mortality are worse and disease incidence is higher, then it can be a bad bargain and may also be producing an inferior end-product. With a smaller unit it is also easier and indeed more likely that better use will be made of the 'waste products', such as manure and litter, because the land nearby may be able to receive it and storage and handling can be kept to a minimum. In future, if the pressure on the need for economy grows as it should, then the highly efficient units must not be so large that they are incapable of giving the best biological results, and are unable to dispose of their waste products easily and usefully.

Environmental control and health

Probably the first group of diseases that comes to mind when considering the relationship between environment and disease is the respiratory complex. It is inevitable that under intensive conditions the likelihood of birds being infected with respiratory ailments is greater than those kept extensively or even semi-intensively. Environmental control has certain major functions. Firstly, it must provide ventilation arrangements that constantly bring in fresh air and draw off stale air, gases and other pollutants. In this way, respiratory by-products that may contain certain disease-producing organisms will be removed. It must, however, perform this vital function in such a way that a uniform movement of the air is applied to the whole area inhabited by the birds, so exchanging the old air with the new in a manner that is virtually imperceptible to the stock. In a later section of this chapter details are given of the practical way in which good ventilation can be achieved, but the reasoning behind the systems should be understood.

As birds are placed in ever greater concentrations it becomes increasingly difficult to get uniform air movement. Far too little attention is given to this and relatively too much to the capacity of the fans, important though the latter may be. It is clear that birds housed intensively do react quite markedly to comparatively minor variations in temperature and air movement, and several studies on the performance of birds in cages have shown that there is a significant difference in various locations, with particular emphasis on the deleterious effects of cold and draughts. At the other end of the scale it is distressing to see heavy mortality occurring in mechanically ventilated poultry houses after sudden rises in the ambient temperature and humidity. To some extent the high mortalities may be due to high stocking densities, but more frequently they seem to have arisen from poor siting and design of the fresh air inlets. Such mortality has occurred even when fan capacities have been more than adequate.

Birds' reaction to illness

When birds become ill with elevated body temperature and reduced appetite and water consumption, they tend to feel the cold more, just as the human subject does when sick. They will then try to congregate, huddling in areas of low air movement. Just how much this aggravates the problem is impossible to say precisely, but it can be surmised that the build-up and intensification of the disease-producing organism is inevitable under the circumstances, causing a vicious circle of yet more disease challenge to the birds. In the case of accommodation where heat is available, a practical procedure is to increase the heat input when the birds are ailing to raise the temperature by several degrees, thus not only tending to persuade the birds to separate one from another but also ensuring that the ventilation rate is not merely maintained but is increased to support any treatment being used. In emphasizing the importance of maintaining warmth to counteract infection, it is also pertinent to stress that many viruses have optimal multiplication temperatures a degree or two below the body temperature of the host so that chilling will promote the harmful effects of these pathogenic organisms.

Control of air movement

It has been stressed that at all times a uniform diffusion of air across the house is essential. There are two quite different ways of achieving this. The most common is to introduce the air into the building at a low speed and either deflect it away with a baffle or diffuse it through slats, perforated inner linings such as slatted hardboard, or media such as mineral, glass wool or canvas. These are frequently used to advantage in 'rescue operations' to diffuse the air into houses with badly designed inlets or to reduce the unfavourable effects of high winds, but they have dangers in that they may reduce the total air entry by restricting the efficiency of fans, or, if they are neglected they may become clogged with dust. Thus they require expert installation and use.

The second approach is to bring the air in at a high velocity and either deflect it abruptly against a baffle-board close to the inlet or direct the air well away from, usually above, the birds so that the draught potential has quite disappeared by the time the air reaches the birds. It is impossible to state categorically which is the best system, and indeed from results in the field it seems that each system, properly designed, can produce equally favourable results. Each form of house seems to have a system most appropriate to its design and use should be made of the right one in assisting to maintain the health of birds. So many houses have a mixture of different systems that no logical pattern can be said to exist, and the essential point to grasp is that most failures occur because they are ill-conceived mixtures of systems.

Another major practical factor in maintaining uniform conditions is the way in which the fans are controlled; there is no need for birds to be subjected to the stress of badly controlled fans. Fans with speed controls enable gentle changes to be made in fan speeds as the climatic conditions change. Most modern arrangements have regulating systems that *gradually* change the speed of the fans and a variable minimum rate can be altered as required according to the age and the stocking rate of the birds. This arrangement is economic where there are large houses requiring a number of fans, but a less sophisticated arrangement may be used satisfactorily with a speed regulator reducing the fan speed to 10% of the maximum. This latter requirement should be specified by the farmer as it is now available on most fans at no extra cost. A unit of two fans, for example one thermostatically controlled and the other on manual regulation, is as good as the most sophisticated system. Indeed it may have certain advantages because it leaves some important functions to the stock-person and does not leave everything to an unfeeling automatic thermostat or thermistor! Recently this type of approach has been more positively advised in multi-fan systems since it requires very simple equipment with little chance of error.

'All-in, all-out' poultry management

Soon after poultry farming entered the era of intensification it was established that there were considerable advantages in following an 'all-in, all-out' programme. This means that all the birds in a unit are housed during the same period, this period being as 'tight' a one as possible and are then taken through to the end of the growing or production period so that the whole unit or site can be cleared of livestock, of all muck, both within and without the houses, and then subsequently disinfected, fumigated and rested for at least a day or two. Such a process has an enormous amount to commend it and the list of advantages given below is impressive.

1. The removal of all living animals off the site can be the biggest factor in eliminating most of the organisms capable of causing disease. The more frequently this 'depopulation' is practised, the more likely it is that any build-up of disease will be prevented.
2. Once the site has been completely cleared of birds it is possible to apply the most rigorous and effective programme of disinfection and fumigation so progressing towards an effective elimination of bacterial, viral, fungal and parasitic infection.
3. The maintenance of birds on a site within a close age range makes for a more uniform state of immunity to disease. Mixed ages lead to an immunological confusion so that the uptake of vaccines or treatment is less satisfactory, and it is much more difficult for the correct administration

of disease prevention programmes as some birds may not respond and/or will receive the treatment at the wrong time.

4. There are sound practical husbandry advantages to filling a site in a single operation. There is only the one unavoidable disturbance and nothing more need be altered until the site is cleared. If units have birds coming and going at irregular intervals, especially introduction of new livestock, the disturbance occurs at various times and can lead to hazards of a health, welfare or behavioural nature.

5. It may also be considered an advantage if the operator can have a pause in the exacting task of management. Maintenance of equipment can also be properly carried out between batches so that there are likely to be fewer breakdowns.

6. In recent years, with the increase in intensification, poultry sites in continuous use have experienced a serious nuisance caused by flies breeding in the manure and other organic matter. Large sites often have poor arrangements for muck disposal. Smells can cause highly objectionable conditions for nearby residents. An 'all-in, all-out' site inevitably limits the feasible size of a unit, which may be considered a good point in itself, but above all it can make it much more practicable to eliminate breeding areas for insects and rodents.

It is emphasized that the merits of depopulation are in inverse proportion to the age of the birds: it is rather less important with the adult because by the time maturity has been reached it may have a satisfactory immunity to most infectious diseases.

Litter management

Management of the 'deep' and 'built-up' litter in a poultry house is of the greatest importance and in practice is one of the most neglected aspects of poultry husbandry. Probably the most serious consequences of bad litter are in breeder houses where wet litter can have a calamitous effect on the feet of the cocks, causing accumulations of infected litter on the feet, subsequently leading to a fall in the level of fertility. In addition the production of clean hatching eggs is impossible.

Good litter needs care—it is not achieved by accident. A start must be made with adequate material, which can be soft wood shavings or chopped straw, although the latter is not advised in the case of breeders for fear of fungal infections. Some poultry farmers use shredded paper, and 'old' litter from previous crops may be used provided it has been completely stacked and heated. A depth of 150 mm at least is required and it should be placed on a dry damp-free base. Studies have shown that litter on an earth base rather than on a damp-proofed concrete floor will contain as much as 10% more moisture on average, so that under these circumstances it may be more difficult, though by no means impossible, to manage. Equally important is the construction of the walls of the house. With an insulated house the insulation must be maintained to the ground.

The ease with which the litter is maintained in a friable state is greatly influenced by the environmental conditions in the house. Uniform temperature and air movement are essential to good litter conditions and an even distribution of birds over the floor; modern systems of air distribution using diffusion of incoming air are capable of giving the best results.

Danger areas in litter management are drinker points, due to splashing, and feeding areas, due to concentration of birds. It may be essential to turn the wet litter quite frequently, and it is often desirable to turn it all from time to time and especially before it is 'working' properly. There is no denying that this is a very laborious task but it can be aided by various mechanical implements which help enormously. Once the litter is working, the activity of the birds themselves will help to keep it in a good condition. The activity benefits the birds, they obtain some nutrients from the litter and the whole atmosphere and environment in the house can be pleasant, not to mention the eventual manurial value of the litter. Working litter is warm and adds warmth to the house, but wet litter is colder and takes heat from the house in an attempt to dry out.

In starting the 'deep litter' house it is better to place a depth of about 70 mm to start with and then add to it as necessary. The smaller the starting depth of litter the more likely the litter is to be totally 'worked' by the birds. Indeed, if a great depth is put in at once the bottom part often is never moved at all through the cycle, especially with broilers, so that its presence is entirely useless and wasteful. By adding litter later, droppings are diluted, the activity of the birds is enhanced, the condition of the litter is improved, and full use of all areas is helped.

When litter is heaped, heated and re-used it is inadvisable to place it in the highly heated brooder area. Firstly, it may present rather too massive a challenge of potentially pathogenic organisms. However, more important is the danger that can result under these circumstances of high levels of ammonia from the warmed litter. High ammonia levels are potentially dangerous for all ages of poultry and they are also most unpleasant for the operator. Levels of up to 15–20 parts per million (ppm) are acceptable. If levels go over 40 ppm there may be some reduction in food intake, but if levels go over 50 ppm the delicate membranes lining the respiratory tract are affected and respiratory disease is much more likely and even blindness can result. By and large it is possible to estimate the levels of ammonia fairly accurately by using one's sense of smell— if it is definitely 'in the air' then it is really too high—but there are more accurate ways of getting an estimate, either by using a litmus paper colour indicator (marketed by Vineland Laboratories) or, more accurately, by using a Draëger gas detector, which can detect levels of a large number of gases by pumping gas, by means of hand bellows, through indicator tubes, which enable an immediate reading to be obtained.

Under the UK's Control of Substances Hazardous to Health Regulations (COSHH) there are maximum levels of dust, put at $10\,mg/m^3$ (inhalable) and $5\,mg/m^3$ (respirable). It is worth bearing in mind that failure to protect workers against the dangers of dust could be grounds for a civil action against the farmer if the worker develops a chest complaint due to negligence. Standards are also laid down for ammonia. The concentration in the air should not exceed 35 ppm if exposure is only for 10 minutes, but if workers are exposed for periods of up to 8 hours the levels must not exceed 25 ppm.

Poultry house construction and insulation

The first need is for a high standard of thermal insulation of surfaces that can be absolutely ensured throughout the period of use of the house. This enables heat conservation to be practised satisfactorily, maintaining the optimum ambient temperature while either eliminating the use of food as a fuel or reducing artificial heat inputs. It also permits a levelling out of any wide diurnal and seasonal temperature variations which may occur and, in association with good ventilation, allows a relative humidity below 80% to be maintained.

The proper way of applying thermal insulation to the buildings is very important but frequently neglected. Many different materials can be used, but it is most essential that these are kept dry. Apart from the fact that many wet materials deteriorate, they also lose their insulating qualities and raise the humidity of the atmosphere. And whilst the importance of weatherproofing is commonly realized, it is not by any means so fully appreciated that it is just as vital to seal the inside from moisture penetration from *within* the building by placing a vapour seal on the warm side of the surface. Suitable vapour seals are polythene, impregnated kraft paper, metal foils and a number of different special paints and liquid sealing compounds. It is also essential to place a damp-proof course at the base of the walls of poultry houses.

Materials that are used for the inside and outside surfaces should be hard-wearing and maintenance-free. For example, a suitable roof construction satisfying all the essential requirements could be made up from the inside to the outside as follows:

1. Flat and rigid fibre boards;
2. A vapour seal of well-lapped polythene sheets;
3. 100–150 mm of glass or mineral wool;
4. An air space giving at least sufficient room to ensure there is no compression of the wool;
5. An outer cladding of corrugated metal.

It is now becoming popular to use an inner lining of polyurethane or polystyrene boards which incorporate suitable vapour seals, either because the substance itself is a barrier or because it incorporates a sealing material on the warm side. Increasing application is being made of forms of polyurethane insulation sprayed on as linings or into cavities to set into a material which is about as hard and as serviceable as the made-up boards.

Similar methods are often followed for the walls, though in this case the outer cladding is more usually of timber for appearance's sake. Whilst timber boards can be used satisfactorily, suitable alternatives are exterior grades of plywood or oil-tempered hardboard. Certain constructions are able to bond the inner cladding, vapour seal and insulation together as, for example, polyurethane faced with aluminium foil or plastic. The final step of bonding the whole wall or roof construction into one piece is actually achieved with the use of polyurethane faced both sides with corrugated steel, aluminium or hardboard usually being used for the exterior surfaces. There seems little doubt that integrated prefabricated processes like this will become increasingly used in poultry house construction and assist the farmer a great deal by giving a clear hygienic surface.

The floor is also of critical importance. Even with a layer of litter, an earth floor can be an obvious place for the build-up of bacteria and parasites. The dangers are greatest to young birds. There is no good alternative to a simple but adequate concrete floor 75–100 mm thick with a damp-proof course between the concrete and the rubble to prevent moisture penetration by capillary attraction from the earth. Careful consideration should be given to the necessary slope of the floor to give good drainage, especially to assist when the building is being cleaned out. In deep-litter systems it is not usually practicable to place drains within the house itself because of blockages, but in cage rearing or laying houses internal drains are of great benefit.

It is likely that within the next few years regulations will emerge that enforce much-improved standards of construction for poultry housing; the main impetus for this will be the demands for impeccable hygiene as an aid to safe eggs and meat. Many existing poultry buildings will become unusable with their porous and damaged surfaces, low standard of thermal insulation and poor environmental control. New buildings required in their place can then provide the very highest standard of thermal insulation, robustness of materials, ease of cleaning and sanitizing, and avoidance of areas where pathogens and their carriers can migrate within their structure (Figures 2.1 & 2.2).

Environmental requirements of poultry

Temperature

Brooding temperatures

A method that is widely used to brood chicks is to arrange a source of warmth in a confined area at about 35 °C (95 °F) at day-old and then subsequently reduce this by 3 °C (5 °F) a week.

To ensure a good use of the house, the house temperature is at least as important as the brooder temperature, a range of 25–30 °C (75–85 °F) being associated with the best all-round performance. Below and above this range weight gains and food conversion efficiencies are reduced. The best performance is usually obtained if the house temperature is reduced from 30 °C (86 °F) during the first week to 27 °C (81 °F) in the second and 24 °C (75 °F) in the third.

If the chicks are to be well distributed within the brooding area the temperature must be uniform and draughts at floor level avoided. Overhead, largely radiant sources of heat give the most satisfactory results since their fine thermostat control and adjustable height offer flexible arrangements. They also serve the dual purpose of brooding and space heating. As an alternative, however, blown hot air has its advocates because of its simplicity, low running costs and good space heating qualities. An initial temperature of 31 °C (88 °F) is recommended in this case which represents something of a compromise between the ideal brooder and house temperature. There should be a reduction of about 0.5 °C (1 °F) daily until a level of 18–21 °C (65–70 °F) is reached. All changes should be made steadily and regularly to avoid stress to the birds.

Post-brooding temperatures

From the age of three weeks onwards some further reductions in temperature are justified. In the case of broilers, the house temperature should be of the order of 18–21 °C (65–70 °F) with a definite tendency to the upper figure if there is any danger of the temperature dropping below 18 °C owing to external conditions. Under ideal conditions the best growth takes place within the range of 18–21 °C and broiler growers should take great care to achieve this

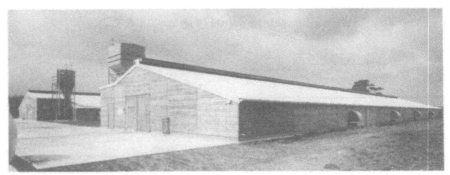

Figure 2.1 Large Controlled Environment Poultry (Broiler) House with side wall extraction enabling foul air to be discharged at or below ground level to minimize spread of disease, dust and smell.

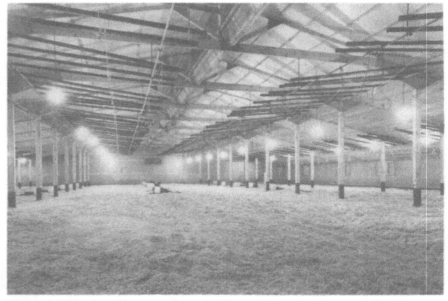

Figure 2.2 Interior of house as shown in Figure 2.1, ready to set up equipment and with soft wood shavings on the floor.

range very gradually, as already mentioned, so that the change is apparently imperceptible to the birds and at the same time ventilation is maintained without a draught. However, in many cases the heat source does not allow the poultry farmer to adjust the temperature so finely or gradually whilst sometimes the ventilation arrangements are inadequate with the higher air velocities demanding a higher temperature to compensate for the cooling effect. Nevertheless, if the ventilation conditions can be maintained satisfactorily, a reduction of some 6 °C (11 °F) between three and nine weeks, giving an eventual temperature of 13–16 °C (55–60 °F) is desirable for optimum growth.

Temperature for layers

For intensively kept birds the optimal temperature is high, i.e. about 21 °C (70 °F). At temperatures below this there is a depression of about ½ egg per hen housed per year per 0.5 °C (1 °F). Feed intake will be reduced by about 7 g per bird per day for a rise from 15 to 21 °C (60 to 70 °F). On the debit side, there is some depression in egg weight, estimated to be about 1 g per egg per 3 °C (6 °F) rise over 15 °C, but this is far outweighed by the benefits. The hen, however, is reasonably adaptable and tolerant to environmental changes and there is a wide range within which it can produce economically even if not at an optimal rate. This range is about 5–24 °C (40–75 °F). However, this does not mean that the temperature can swing rapidly between these two extremes since rapid changes of any sort are undesirable. Rather it represents the seasonal extremes one should aim for in designing housing for less intensive systems, such as deep-litter and the strawyard. Provided the changes take place gradually, birds can acclimatize to them.

If the temperature rises above 24 °C for lengthy periods the total number of eggs laid and their weight and quality will certainly suffer. Appetite will also fall. Below 5 °C the chief effect will be a sharply rising appetite, though egg weight and quality can benefit slightly. It may be possible to compensate for the failing appetite at high temperatures by increasing the essential nutrients in the ration and so produce as many eggs of almost as good quality on a reduced and hence more economical quantity of food.

In order to obtain the required temperature conditions in a temperate climate such as the UK's, it is usual to rely upon an excellent standard of thermal insulation and controlled ventilation.

Humidity

There is no reason to have a firmly set range for the humidity of the air though in practical terms the aim in the winter months will be to keep the relative humidity below about 80% of saturation and preferably nearer to a maximum of 75%. Normally there need be no problems with chickens if the relative humidity is low, but this is not true if the birds are suffering from respiratory disease; the evidence is that humidities below 50% and especially as low as 30%, may to some extent aggravate infection and help contagion. Infectious particles stay suspended and viable for longer periods in dry, dusty air. It is mainly for this reason that higher ventilation rates are advised for summer nowadays because whilst it is not usually practicable to consider humidifying the air to deal with this problem, the dilution of infection and prevention of high dust content of the atmosphere can be dealt with indirectly by high air change rates.

Water cooling

Problems sometimes occur in temperate climates, and often in hot climates, of buildings becoming overheated either momentarily or for quite long periods. This may sometimes arise from poor thermal insulation of the building or there may be insufficient fans or they may be operating inefficiently. If these obvious faults cannot be corrected, or in cases where after this it is still too warm, there are several ways of using water to cool the building.

A simple device is to spray water over the roof and walls, thereby cooling by evaporation; in some cases a perforated waterpipe is placed along the roof ridge to discharge water uniformly along the length of the roof. A more usual way is to pass the incoming air through wet pads; the pads may consist of a wooden frame filled with absorbent wood fibres with water falling through from top to bottom. Surplus water has to be collected and recirculated to be economical, and the pads must be kept clean if they are to function successfully.

A still better way is to have spray nozzles which produce a very fine mist.

A fourth and perhaps the best method of all consists of a metal disc revolving at high speed which throws off water onto an atomizing plate which sets up a very fine mist taken up by the airstream. Good control is achievable by a solenoid valve activated by a humidistat.

Lighting requirements

The development of the reproductive (egg-laying) organ is stimulated by increasing amounts of daylight, as in spring, but is depressed when this is reduced as in autumn. The modern genetically improved layer, under the stimulus of spring-like conditions, will lay before sufficient bodily development has taken place to fully support egg production and it will be incapable of laying either the number or size of eggs achievable in later life. An autumn-like pattern, or even a constant day length, will allow the body to develop properly before the bird starts laying. Thereafter to stimulate maximum production, the procedure is to give a weekly increase of light duration of about 20 minutes up to a maximum of 16 to 18 hours. Artificial lighting is of course essential if this is to be achieved at all seasons, though by rearing chicks in the autumn the natural advantage of seasonal changes can be exploited.

A number of techniques are used in order to get the most favourable response, and although most are rather similar each breeder tends to suggest something different for his own stock, based on sound practical experience. Two programmes are given below for a well-known commercial hybrid. It is noteworthy that the maximum amount of light in one day is given as 18 hours.

A suggested lighting programme for commercial hybrid layers is:

0–1 week	18 hours light, 6 hours darkness
2–18 weeks	6 hours light, 18 hours darkness
19–22 weeks	Increase light by 45 minutes per week to give a good stimulus at the first period of laying
23–49 weeks	Increase light by 20 minutes per week
49 weeks onwards	Lighting kept steady at 18 hours light per day

Those retailing eggs and seeking especially large eggs can use the following variant:

0–1 week	23 hours light
2–18 weeks	Decrease by 45 minutes per week
19–22 weeks	Increase by 45 minutes per week
23–48 weeks	Increase by 20 minutes per week
49 weeks onwards	Retain at 18 hours of light

A more recent technique is the use of ahemeral lighting cycles. These are daily light cycles greater or less than 24 hours. These are not capable of altering egg output, but they can improve egg weight and shell strength so that there can be economic advantage to the farmer if prices for larger eggs are suitably favourable. The number of second quality eggs can also be reduced. A 28-hour light cycle which uses bright and then dimmed lights has real advantages. The dim lights enable egg collections and stock inspections at any time even during the birds' 'night' period; the bright lights have 30 times more intensity than the dim and this stimulates 'day' (bright) and 'night' (dim). A suitable ahemeral lighting programme as devised by the Poultry Department of the North of Scotland College of Agriculture is shown in Figure 2.3.

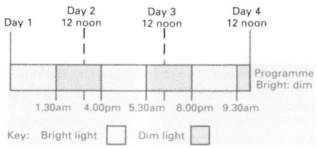

Figure 2.3 Chart showing lighting programme for 28-hour ahemeral light cycle.

For broilers the usual pattern throughout most of the industry is to have 23 hours lighting and 1 hour darkness in each 24 hours, the latter being necessary to train the birds to darkness. If this is not done and the light is suddenly withdrawn for some reason, a pile-up is a likely consequence, the birds tending to crowd into corners and suffocate.

There is, however, an increasing interest now in growing broilers under intermittent lighting patterns, which were once popular; these appear capable of some improvement in growth rate but more particularly in the food conversion ratio. They are capable of improving digestion with suitable rest periods, decreasing activity and reducing 'boredom eating'. A suitable lighting pattern is as follows:

0–3 weeks	Continuous lighting (with 1 hour off in 24)
3–5 weeks cycle	3 hours on and 1 hour off
5–7 weeks cycle	2 hours on and 2 hours off
7 weeks onwards cycle	1 hour on and 3 hours off

Continuous lighting for broilers can be with a light intensity as low as 0.2 lux, which is about as low as the 'off' phase in a controlled environment house in the daytime.

Lighting procedure

For proper artificial control of lighting, exclusion of all natural light must be complete. Fully efficient baffles under fan shafts or in air inlet hoods and around the edges of the ventilators are essential. The insides of the ventilators should be painted black. The maximum safe level of intensity of stray light entering houses which are supposed to be blacked out is 0.4 lux and it is advisable if there are any doubts on this score to check the intensity using a light meter. For stimulation of layers the light intensity should be 10–16 lux and there is no advantage from raising the level above this.

If light intensity is uneven in the house, with bright and dark areas, the birds will favour and concentrate in certain areas. This will tend to cause the development of vices and diseases, particularly respiratory ones. In every poultry house lighting circuit a dimming device is necessary, so that light intensity can be lowered easily should there be an outbreak of cannibalism. If birds are to receive sufficient and even light intensity, the disposition of the light must be uniform. This uniformity is usually obtained by suspending ordinary tungsten bulbs at about 3 m (10 ft) centres along and across the house. A reflector over the bulb will assist in maintaining an even intensity and will help to keep the bulbs free of settled dust.

Suitable systems of lighting are now marketed which utilize fluorescent lighting tubes with dimming arrangements and whilst the capital cost of these is somewhat greater than tungsten bulbs, their increased efficiency enables a substantial saving in running costs which can soon recoup the higher initial charge.

Ventilation

Ventilation is concerned with almost all the individual items of the climatic environment, or strictly, the microclimate. It must eliminate the by-products of respiration and excretion of the bird, and evaporates from the droppings and its litter. It is also concerned with the control of temperature in the house and humidity as emphasized earlier. Also, it has to change the air within the building so that the speed of air movement is uniform throughout the house. Considerable variation is required from winter to summer (Table 2.1). In winter a speed of 0.15–0.25 m/s (30–50 ft/min) is correct, whereas in summer a movement of at least five or six times that figure is called for.

Table 2.1 Guiding standards for ventilation rates in poultry houses

Season	Ventilation rate (m³/h/kg body weight)	
	Broilers	Adults
Summer/maximum	4.0	8.0
Winter/minimum	0.7	1.5

Most of the modern developments in intensive poultry management have been concentrated on the so-called controlled-environment house, though it is frequently emphasized that such control as this title implies is but rarely achieved. A controlled-environment house regulates the ambient temperature, air movement, ventilation and light (see Figure 2.1). The standard of construction, thermal insulation and ventilation must be high but the cost per bird is brought down to an economic level by stocking at a relatively high density. High densities of stock put a very great burden on the ventilation and the design skill required to achieve all these aims must be very high. Ventilation rates are given below and reference should be made to these for the required figures.

Practical ventilation

Ventilation systems should be kept simple and easy for the stockperson to control. Arrangements must always be available for a system that will function should the fans or electricity fail, either by designing it so that natural convection can take over temporarily, or by the provision of an alternative emergency power supply.

The incoming air must reach the birds at a low velocity in the cold weather; it should also be at the ambient air temperature when it moves over the birds, at which time a uniform air velocity should be maintained. This last point is important to ensure an even distribution of birds on the floor, particularly if they are already stocked at a maximum density.

With ridge extraction systems an inlet velocity of 60 m/min (200 ft/min) is achieved by allowing 0.5 m^2 (5 ft^2) of inlet area for each 1700 m^3/hour (1000 ft^3/min) extracted. The air inlet velocity is possibly even more important than the air inlet direction, but where the air comes in at the sides of the house the direction of entry should be controllable, and when the ambient air outside is cooler than that inside, the air should always be directed upwards away from the floor. If the air enters under the direct pressure of the fans, baffle arrangements should be incorporated to deflect it from causing direct draughts on the stock. If these requirements are carefully attended to, inlet areas as low as 0.18 m^2/1700 m^3/h (2 ft^2/1000 ft^3/min) are perfectly satisfactory.

The air should enter or leave the house evenly around the walls or along its length; there must be no dead spots created by large gaps between the ventilators.

The ventilation system should be able to cope in a semi-automatic way with the extremely wide range between maximum and minimum ventilation requirements, a ratio of up to approximately 100 to 1. For example, in a broiler house where a finished bird requires 7 m^3 of fresh air/hour in summer, a day-old chick in winter requires no more than 0.08 m^3/hour.

In order to obtain the fine control required, it is usual to have a number of fans and speed controls. Thus the fans in use may be progressively increased in number and speed from the minimum demands needed for the young chick. There are a number of acceptable arrangements to choose from; the important features to look for are speed control of all fans and independent operation of individual, or groups, of fans. With multi-fan systems it is possible with certain designs to avoid using speed regulators by the use of controls that switch the fans on and off in series. The great advantage of such systems is that they are less costly to buy, reliable, cheap to run, and efficient.

Ventilation systems

The simplest arrangement is to have hopper inlet openings situated along the walls of the building. These are bottom-hinged and open between gussets. The outer hood, with a light and wind baffle, is an essential part. On exposed sites the benefits of the baffle in helping to overcome the effects of strong winds is considerable, and is worth incorporating even when the need for such fine light control is not indicated. Figures 2.4 and 2.5 illustrate two types of baffle.

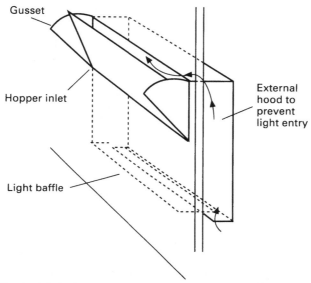

Figure 2.4 Fresh air inlet incorporating hopper and wind and light traps.

An alternative, more advanced, arrangement is shown in Figure 2.6. This shows a louvered intake which is set in the inner part of the wall so that there is no obstruction. The louvers give complete directional control which can be arranged from a limited number of points. Automatic regulation is also feasible. Instead of a projecting hood, the air enters the space between inner and outer linings at the base of the wall. This means a tidier appearance, less maintenance and better elimination of light and the unfavourable effects of wind.

Another arrangement is the high-speed inlet jet system. The principle of this is to design the inlets so that the incoming air is drawn in at high speed— usually under the ceiling or roof, which must be unobstructed. This airstream sets up a number of secondary circular currents of gentle movement which actually ventilate the birds. The advantages are that the small inlet assists in reducing the wind's unfavourable effect on ventilation thereby ensuring that the air movement and distribution are uniform, stable and predictable. Inlet speeds at the intake are usually maintained at least at 5 m/s (1000 ft/min). New

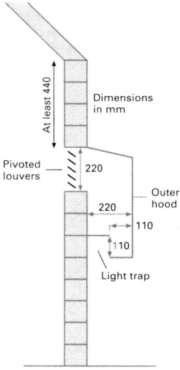

Figure 2.5 An alternative arrangement of air inlet for controlled-environment housing.

control devices have been designed to give automatic regulation of the inlet area and the number of fans operating which must be at full speed or 'off'. This system gives very economical control and is an energy conserver by utilizing a minimum number of fans at top speed and by keeping the coolest air under the ceiling surfaces.

Extracting fans are usually placed in the ridge. Manufacturers' cowls can be used but, as they are rather expensive, the more usual procedure is to place the fan in a square timber trunk. The trunk should be larger in area than the fan, but a diaphragm fitting round the blades is vital. A light trap is needed underneath and the cap over the top also has a lip to assist in keeping light out. Typical dimensions are shown in Figure 2.7. A chimney trunk of 750 mm × 750 mm (30 in × 30 in) is used for a 600 mm (24 in) diameter fan. The fan is placed at the base of the trunk in its diaphragm plate—this is, in fact, the most efficient placing and it is also easiest for maintenance. If there is a power failure, the trunks serve as straightforward static extractors and save the house from becoming disastrously hot and under-ventilated. In any sizeable unit a

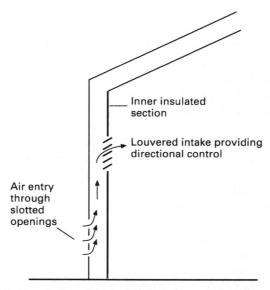

Figure 2.6 An excellent design of fresh air inlet integrated into the wall structure.

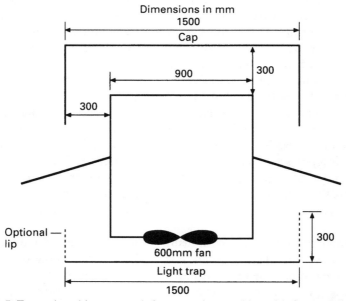

Figure 2.7 Extracting chimney trunk for mounting on ridge with fans and light trap.

stand-by generator is best to cope with power failure and with most other systems of ventilation it is an essential part of the enterprise.

The conventional system of ventilation described here remains suitable for buildings up to about 16 m (50 ft) span. The system is suitable for birds in tiered cages when up to three rows are used. However, with four or more rows, the outer cages tend to produce a barrier preventing air from reaching the centre and make additional inlets necessary. One way of providing them is either to place ducts under the floor to open under the central cages, or to raise the whole floor off the ground so the air can enter under the central rows. Alternatively, ceiling inlets by strip-gaps or areas of glass-fibre which bring air down between the central rows can be installed. Yet a third arrangement has been used very successfully in cage laying houses of up to approximately 30 m (100 ft) in length with the air being blown from end to end. It is pertinent to emphasize that in all cage laying houses a satisfactory air flow is more likely to result if the passages between the cages are adequate. A 1.3 m (4 ft) passageway is ideal in this respect.

In certain cases, such as wide-span houses and deep-pit houses with stair-step (Californian) or flat-deck cages, the air is brought in through the ridge and extracting fans may be placed in the wall. The design of the inlet at the ridge is of great importance to prevent cold down-draughts on the birds. One way of avoiding the draughts is to place inlet chimneys in the roof with the air passing into them at not more than 243 m/min (800 ft/min) (inlet area about 0.054 m^2 (1.5 ft^2) per 1700 m^3/h (1000 ft^3/min) extracted.

An alternative arrangement is to use an open ridge with a baffle board underneath; this may be fixed in position, which is a simple, unsophisticated arrangement, or may be controlled both in area and direction so that different degrees of opening and alternative arrangements for the deflection of the air can be achieved. Such controls may be automatic machine-operated (Figure 2.8). Downturned fan boxes, as shown in Figure 2.9, may be protected from the adverse effect of the wind by the use of a suitable windbreak.

In any system of poultry housing where the droppings accumulate under the birds, such as the deep-pit house, it is absolutely essential to have a reversed flow with the air passing in at the ridge or ceiling, then to the birds and finally over the droppings and out. This keeps the air purer and free of gases, and the droppings dry more quickly. Whilst it is still common practice to achieve this by placing the extraction fans in the pit area, it is now becoming more popular to pressurize the house and place the fans on the input side to create the pressure.

A warning must be given. With many of the most sophisticated mechanical ventilation systems, if there is any failure in electrical supply or fan break-down, there can be little or no air flow. Thus there is a grave risk of the birds suffocating. Measures must be taken to install an alarm to warn of failure, and a stand-by generator to take over if there is an interruption of mains supply. In

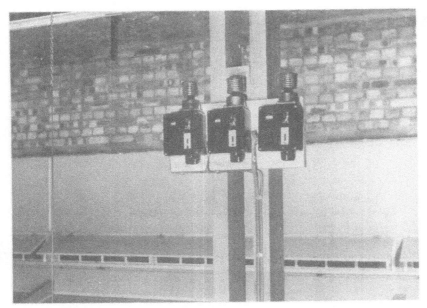

Figure 2.8 Thermostatic motorized controls used for automatic control of mechanical or natural ventilation.

the absence of a generator, a fail-safe system should be provided in which a considerable area of shutters, normally held together by electromagnets, can open automatically when the electric current fails. Great care is needed in making such provisions and expert advice should be sought for the installation of alarms, generators and fail-safe measures. It is mandatory to install such systems in the UK.

Natural ventilation

Quite recently there has been renewed interest in natural ventilation systems relying entirely on natural convection and air flow. These have much to commend them if it is accepted that stocking densities must be reduced and management will need to be more careful and even meticulous in its attention. The arrangements are described in some detail in the section on poultry management in hot climates later in this chapter.

An additional arrangement now becoming popular in the UK is that known as automatically controlled natural ventilation (ACNV) whereby the area of opening of both inlets and outlets is controlled by motors activated by thermostats or occasionally additionally by humidistats.

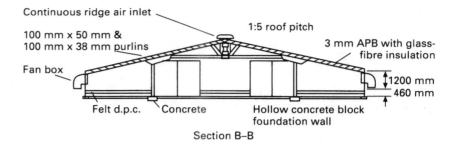

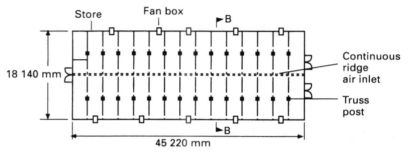

Figure 2.9 Ridge inlet system with wall extracting fans.

Disinfection of poultry houses

Natural disinfecting agents

The survival of avian pathogens outside the animal body varies considerably depending on the species of the agent and whether it is protected with organic matter; for example, the spores of bacteria can remain viable virtually indefinitely in the soil or protected in cracks and crevices of a building.

The factors contributing towards the natural destruction of pathogens are important as they reduce the environmental burden. They include sunlight, heat, cold, desiccation and agitation. Sunlight is the most potent and its powers of destruction are enormous due to the ultraviolet range of wavelengths. Unfortunately these ultraviolet rays have little penetrating power and cannot pass through glass, translucent roofing sheets or dust. The value of sunlight within poultry buildings is therefore almost nil, but it is an important factor in the surrounding area. Desiccation from fresh air and wind will also contribute to pathogen destruction, particularly when the microorganisms are exposed to this by prior cleansing of the building.

Another process is antibiosis. Many bacteria and fungi produce substances which are antagonistic to other organisms. Penicillin and streptomycin are such substances whose antibacterial action is well known. In the soil, in floors and buildings generally, pathogenic organisms will be acted upon by anti-biotics produced by non-pathogenic organisms which may be found in poultry houses. Warm, moist conditions will assist the action of such saprophytic agents.

The action of heat

For many years heat has been used for disinfection, dry heat being used with the 'flame-gun' and moist heat in the form of the 'steam-jenny', but both tend to be inexact and are sometimes dangerous and uncontrollable methods of applying the agents.

Many bacterial spores can easily survive the transitory attention of the heat source and pathogenic organisms may readily be protected from the heat in cracks and crevices of the building.

Chemical disinfectants and disinfection

Disinfection on the farm is generally carried out by using chemical agents (Figure 2.10). The lethal action of disinfectants is due in the main to their ability to react with the protein and, in particular, the essential enzymes of microorganisms. Therefore any agent that will coagulate, precipitate or other-wise denature proteins will act as a general disinfectant. Among these agents are phenols, alcohols, acids, alkalis, aldehydes, halogens, chloramines and quaternary ammonium compounds.

Selective action

Many disinfectants have a selective action on different types of microbes depending on the stucture of the organisms; for example, Gram-positive and Gram-negative bacteria differ in the structure of their cell walls and react quite differently.

It is also vital to stress that disinfection is not an instantaneous matter—it takes place gradually. However, many more microbes are killed at the begin-ning of the process than at the end although there is an initial lag period before activity commences. An examination of the number of organisms surviving at different stages during disinfection shows that the number of bacteria killed in unit time bears a constant relationship to the number of surviving organisms. Thus, after an initial lag phase, destruction of the pathogens is very rapid at first but tends to slow up so that eventually destruction of all the organisms takes a considerably longer time. It requires emphasis that disinfectants must

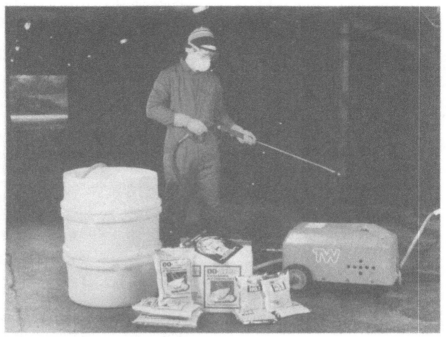

Figure 2.10 Power washing a poultry house.

be given time to inactivate microorganisms, which means in practice a period of some 24 hours.

The concentration of disinfectant and temperature of disinfectant influence the rate of death and also alter the shape of time–survivor curves. As the death rate is increased by using higher concentrations of disinfectant, the initial lag phase is eliminated or is so short that it goes undetected.

The activity of most disinfectants improves markedly if the temperature is increased; many of the common mild disinfectants are relatively ineffective at temperatures near freezing. The 'temperature coefficient' is the measure of the change in velocity of disinfection per degree rise in temperature:

$$\text{Temperature coefficient (per } 10° \text{ rise)} = \frac{\text{Time to kill at } x°}{\text{Time to kill at } (x + 10°)}$$

The coefficient is an exponential factor, as is the dilution coefficient. The effect of dilutions, however, varies widely between disinfectants. For example, phenolic substances are considerably affected, so the coefficient is high.

The effect of organic matter

Almost invariably when disinfection is carried out on the poultry farm organic matter will be present. This seriously interferes with the action of the disinfectant in the following ways:

1. The organic matter may protect the cell by forming a coating on it and preventing the ready access of the disinfectant.
2. The disinfectant may form an insoluble compound with the organic matter to remove it from potential activity.
3. The disinfectant may react chemically with the organic matter giving rise to a non-germicidal reaction product.
4. Particulate and colloidal matter in suspension may absorb the anti-bacterial agent, so that it is substantially removed from solution.
5. Fats may inactivate the disinfectant.

Cleaning before the application of the disinfectant is essential and the process is aided by the availability of very efficient combined detergent disinfectants.

Types of disinfectants

The phenols and related compounds comprise one of the most important groups of disinfectants, acting bactericidally or fungicidally, though being poorly sporicidal and virucidal. They have high dilution coefficients, i.e. small changes in concentration give rise to large differences in their killing rates, and they are always more effective as the temperature rises and are more active as acid solutions. Organic matter severely interferes with their efficiency. There are many 'coal-tar disinfectants', phenolic in nature, and in view of their inevitable low solubility in water, they are either solubilized or emulsified. The soluble types, known as 'black fluids', are those in which the phenol fraction is dissolved in a soap base; the emulsified types, known as the 'white fluids', are those in which the phenol is emulsified into a permanent suspension with the aid of gelatin or dextrin. Both are widely used in and around poultry buildings.

In more recent years a number of synthetic phenols have been marketed. Such preparations are non-toxic, non-irritant and a more pleasant odour, arising chiefly from their purer nature. They have limited use in poultry husbandry as they are essentially for domestic use and are both expensive and easily inactivated.

Oxidizing agents

Hydrogen peroxide and other oxidizing agents, including peracetic and propionic acids and acid peroxygen systems, are emerging as increasingly popular disinfectants. At quite low concentrations they are active against bacteria, bacterial spores, viruses and fungi. Several new and safe proprietary forms are available for use in poultry houses.

The halogens

In agriculture, chlorine is widely used for disinfecting water and in the cleansing of equipment. Chlorine-releasing compounds containing up to 90% available chlorine are available and have an important use in the formulation of bactericidal detergent powders of the alkaline variety. Products of this type are suitable for use in the washing down of poultry buildings. The inorganic chloramines, being a concentration of chlorine and ammonia, are used in water and sewage treatment, as are organic chloramines such as halazone, which is an excellent water sanitizer.

Failure of chlorine disinfection is most likely due to the presence of organic matter, which seriously interferes with its action so that it is not normally used where much dirt is present.

Iodine is an effective germicide although, like chlorine, its action is greatly depressed by organic matter. It is effective against vegetative organisms and spores. The most widely used iodine preparations are the iodophors in which iodine is mixed with surface-active agents, which act as carriers or solubilizers for the iodine. They lack any real odour and are not irritant.

Iodophors are an ideal germicide to use in water utensils. When formulated with certain acids they are effective against a wide variety of bacterial and viral pathogens of poultry.

Ammonia

A 10% aqueous solution of ammonia is an effective agent for the destruction of coccidial oocysts. This is the only use for ammonia as a disinfectant. Proprietary disinfectants are available which combine ammonia-releasing compounds with general disinfectants. Personnel using these must wear protective masks.

Quaternary ammonium compounds

Quaternary ammonium compounds are cationic neutral detergents available as aqueous solutions, powders or pastes. They are effective against a wide range of bacteria and moulds and have a high surface activity. Generally, when dissolved in water, they have a high wetting power and the ions adhere to surfaces giving a long-lasting residual effect. They also have low toxicity and lack odour or taste. Combined with other disinfectants they can give a wide spectrum of activity.

Gaseous and aerosol fumigation

The use of gases and vapours for disinfection is increasing in popularity. They usually do little or no harm to the materials used in the construction of the house, or to the electrical and heating installation. It is also comparatively simple for any disinfecting gas to be removed from the house after use. Gases are toxic to humans, so great care must always be taken in their use and safety regulations rigidly followed.

Formaldehyde has been used for many years as a comprehensive fumigant. All bacteria, including spores, are susceptible to formaldehyde gas even in the presence of some organic matter, so it is clearly the type of material to use for general purposes. It may be used in a number of ways. A popular way is by the interaction of formalin and potassium permanganate: 80 ml of formalin to $10 \, m^3$ for buildings up to $1000 \, m^3$, and 40 ml per $10 \, m^3$ for larger buildings up to $2000 \, m^3$. The ratio of permanganate to formalin required for optimal generation of formaldehyde is 2 parts permanganate to 3 parts formalin. Great care must be taken in this operation as the compounds react with violence. No more than 1 litre of formalin should be put into each container, which should have deep sides to prevent the mixture bubbling over. As there is a risk of fire, litter and wooden members of the house should be kept out of range. The operator should wear a respirator while carrying out the procedure.

Formaldehyde gas may also be released from solid paraformaldehyde which can be placed on remote-controlled electric hot plates at a rate of 1 kg per $300 \, m^3$ (2.2 lb per $10\,600 \, ft^3$) of building. For optimum results the building should be warmed to 20 °C (68 °F) or above; many failures are recorded when reliance has been placed on formaldehyde at cold winter temperatures in the order of 0–10 °C (32–50 °F).

An alternative means of fumigating buildings is to disperse a mixture of formalin and water as an aerosol of small particle size, at the rate of 30–60 ml to each $6-10 \, m^3$ ($200-350 \, ft^3$) of air space. The higher the humidity the better it works, 60–80% being considered the optimum. The space to be fumigated should be kept sealed and closed for at least 12 hours.

Formaldehyde is undoubtedly the best terminal disinfectant. It is sometimes difficult to remove after use owing to the fact that the formaldehyde does not remain in gaseous form during sterilization, but becomes absorbed on exposed surfaces as a film of polymerized formaldehyde; this may be dealt with by sprinkling a weak solution of ammonia in the house.

As an alternative to formaldehyde alone a highly active complex disinfectant which is useful against the most persistent viruses is one containing formaldehyde, glutaraldehyde and a quaternary ammonium compound. This is active at much lower temperatures than formaldehyde.

Aerosols

Aerosol particles consist of suspensions of solid or liquid particles in the atmosphere which are of a size less than 200 μm diameter and in this form they remain in suspension for a considerable time. Their lightness enables them to flow over and around any solid objects and they can penetrate behind equipment and divisions. High-velocity generators can be used to distribute disinfectants within a few minutes in buildings as large as $1000 \, m^3$ ($35\,000 \, ft^3$) capacity even from a single point. This dispersibility of aerosols can be used to provide either an even distribution of vapour in the atmosphere or an even deposition of a film of disinfectant on horizontal and vertical surfaces. This may be used either for disinfection of the air when the animals are in occupation or for terminal disinfection when the building is empty.

Ectoparasites and insects

It is of great importance to control ectoparasites in and around the poultry houses. They are a nuisance both to the attendants and the birds; they may be the cause of direct irritation and disease, and they may indirectly spread disease; indeed, any infectious agent can be carried by ectoparasitic vectors. These ectoparasites include flies (the common house-fly, the lesser house-fly and the stable-fly), mites (red mites and northern fowl mites), ticks, lice, fleas, bugs and beetles and cockroaches.

For the control of external parasites of animals several compounds are available, such as gamma benzene hexachloride (Lindane), piperoxyl-butoxide pyrethrum (Pybuthrin) or 0 0-dimethyldithiophosphate of diethylmercaptosuccinate (Malathion) and 0 0-dimethyl 0,245 trichlorphenyl phosphorathroate (Fenchlorphos 12%). Products are marketed in a number of forms including liquids for spraying or for mixing into the litter, or as paints for perches and wooden parts of the house, or for direct application to birds (Figure 2.11).

One of the greatest problems in the controlled environment poultry house arises from the lesser mealworm beetle (*Alphitobius diaperinus*). It is extremely persistent as it tends to maintain an existence between crops by retreating into the fabric of the house and emerging safely from this protected environment after the disinfecting process. It has been shown positively to act as a carrier for the following diseases, amongst others: mycotoxicosis, leucosis, Marek's disease, salmonellosis, colibacillosis. The only solution is to give repeated applications of an insecticide, choosing one with penetrating and residual activity. The beetle has a life cycle of a minimum of about 28 days and the reproductive

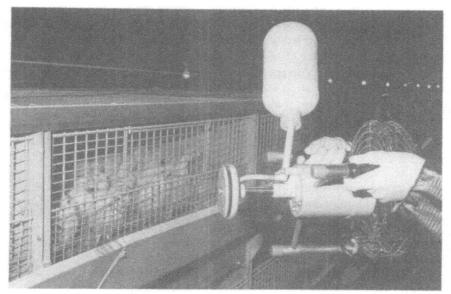

Figure 2.11 Insecticide application to birds in cages using a product approved for direct application.

rate is enormous under warm and humid conditions which are common in poultry houses.

Disposal of carcases and litter

Ideally carcases are disposed of on the site. Incineration is the best method, but is expensive and not always practicable. An alternative is to have a purpose-made deep burial pit, which is covered and is also approved by the local authority and the water and drainage authorities in order to ensure there is no danger of contamination of water courses or supplies. In practice carcases are often removed from the site and either safely disposed of elsewhere or made use of by maggot breeders. In such cases the carcases should be carefully placed in sealed and airtight polythene bags and placed in a safe collection point, but outside the security of the site to reduce any disease risk from the collection lorry, which may contain other carcases. A regular collection is essential—rotting carcases present a considerable risk of disease spread and may be attacked by vermin. A sealed container or skip is desirable for their storage. Regrettably the handling of mortality on poultry sites is rarely given the attention it deserves nor are the enormous risks of bad handling fully comprehended. Much the same may be said of the dangers of the litter taken from poultry houses after the flock has been depopulated.

In recent virulent epidemics of infectious bursal disease, outbreaks of the disease appeared to be promoted rapidly through the spreading of litter taken from infected houses. In many cases seen by the author, the disease occurred almost immediately after (1–4 days) infected litter was spread on adjoining fields. To avoid such occurrences, litter and manure after removal from a site should be taken to a location well away from any poultry sites and stacked for 3–6 months. It would be a wise precaution to spray the outside of the heap with disinfectant, and if at all possible protect it from any wildlife that may spread infection.

Recommended procedure in disinfection and disinfestation of poultry buildings and equipment

Basically two procedures should be adopted, the first being that used between batches of poultry within a building in the absence of overt disease, and the second after outbreaks of contagious and infectious diseases.

Procedure of disinfection with no known disease present

1. All equipment and fittings that are removable should be taken out of the building and then soaked in a bath of disinfectant, or power-sprayed or steam sterilized.
2. All litter should be removed.
3. The roof and structural elements of the house should be dusted and cleaned, preferably with a vacuum cleaner.
4. The lower part of the walls and all the floors should be thoroughly cleaned—preferably using a pressure washer—with a heavy-duty, wide-spectrum detergent-disinfectant mixture.
5. The surfaces must then have a disinfectant applied with a wide spectrum of activity, capable of killing all types of pathogens present.
6. In certain cases, if there is a heavy insect infestation, there will be a need to apply a special insecticide spray.
7. As a final measure the building may be gassed with formaldehyde or with a disinfectant to give a residual effect. Thermal 'fogging' machines are widely used.

Procedure after contagious and infectious disease

1. The building should be closed and isolated from all visitors.
2. The bedding, litter and all areas in intimate contact with the birds should be sprayed with a disinfectant at adequate concentration.

3. The litter should subsequently be removed from the building and may be burnt or buried so there is no possible contact with poultry or other livestock.
4. Portable equipment and fittings should be given the same treatment and preferably in the house, later to be taken out and aerated.
5. The floors and lower part of the walls are treated with a detergent-disinfectant.
6. The house should then be treated in the same way as suggested in the previous section.
7. It may sometimes be advisable to skim off the top few inches of the soil around a heavily infected area.
8. The approaches to the building should be treated with disinfectant; foot-dips should be provided for personnel and wheel-dips for vehicles.

Possible sources of public nuisance from poultry units

In recent years there have been increasing objections from residents near poultry sites claiming that they suffer nuisance from smell, dust, flies and noise. It is claimed that this is not only destructive to the quality of their lives but also causes ill-health. Though many of the complaints are ill-founded, everything should be done to reduce the possibilities of these nuisances and the following measures may help towards this end.

It is preferable for a mechanical ventilation system to have a positive wall extraction arrangement discharging the foul air downwards onto the ground (see Figure 2.1). To further reduce the spread of smell and dust the extracted air can be dischargd onto a sump containing disinfectant and deodorant with a hessian curtain protecting the area of discharge (Figure 2.12). Placing the fans on the walls also reduces the possibility of noise, which can be further reduced with sound insulation panels placed in the hood; in addition, special fan mountings will help further to reduce any risk of noise.

When litter or muck are removed the loaded trailer should be covered before moving off the site and the contents taken far away from any danger of causing smell to neighbouring residents.

Good ventilation and environmental conditions will greatly help in reducing smell. One of the least pleasant manifestations is the smell that arises from extremely damp litter in the terminal stages of a broiler crop and when this is being cleared. Good temperature and ventilation, no overstocking, proper choice and management of drinkers to reduce spillage and good management

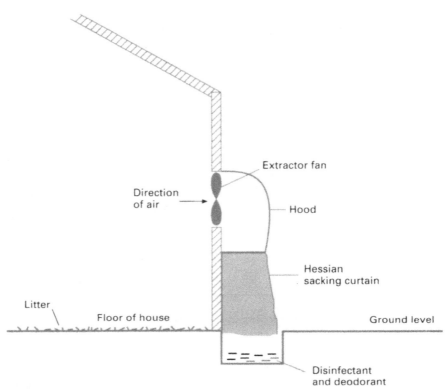

Figure 2.12 Ventilation extraction to reduce dust and smells.

of litter will assist greatly. Many of the complaints that arise from nearby residents are magnified if such care is not taken.

One of the greatest aids in reducing smell is to plant a belt of trees between the poultry site and the houses. The trees assist by trapping the dust and smell and also isolating the site from cross-winds. Also it helps psychologically if the site cannot be seen.

The flies which may be associated with some sites are due to lack of attention to the cleanliness of the poultry houses and their surroundings which thereby afford breeding areas for the flies. The whole of the site should be kept in the same good order as the houses and herbage cut or land cultivated. Flies may also breed in the dung in deep pit houses, and this may need to be treated with insecticide to prevent this.

Litter condition has also been improved by the addition of zeolites, which are crystalline hydrated aluminosilicates of alkaline earth cations. These have the ability to absorb and control the amount of ammonia and moisture and thereby reduce the nuisance but, in addition, they have beneficial effects on growth and egg production and reduce the amount of foot pad burns. There are other additives to litter that make similar claims but they are not widely used due to their expense. Good management of the environment is above all the best way to reduce complaints of manure smells.

Management of poultry in hot climates

Large poultry units are increasingly being established in countries with hot climates, where advanced methods of husbandry are a recent introduction. Special techniques should be considered for the satisfactory management of birds under these conditions.

Housing and environment

Naturally ventilated (or convection housing)

There is no firm agreement amongst experts as to whether it is preferable to have open types of freely ventilated natural convection housing or controlled environment housing in hot climates (Plates 1 and 2). My own preference is to use naturally ventilated housing with relatively light stocking densities wherever there are doubts about the reliability of the power supply, or the management skills are relatively unsophisticated. Buildings such as those shown in Figures 2.13 and 2.14 will give ideal conditions in most warm climates and

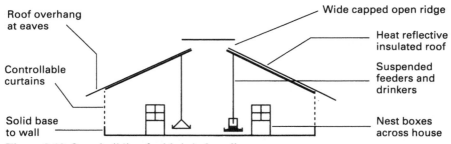

Figure 2.13 Span building for birds in hot climates.

there is a great facility for variation in the amount of ventilation and air movement by the use of controllable curtains at the front or sides of the building. This is generally essential as diurnal variation in temperature and air movement can be very great in tropical climates.

In nearly all circumstances it is desirable that the roof of the building is

57

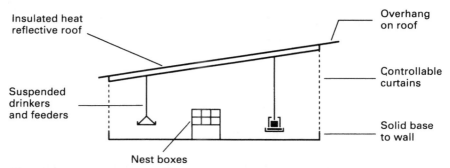

Figure 2.14 Monopitch building for birds in hot climates.

insulated to a high standard, equivalent to about 150 mm (6 in) of glass fibre or 100 mm (4 in) of expanded plastic. The outer claddings should be in light heat reflective materials.

The width of naturally ventilated houses should not exceed 13 m (40 ft), and the ridge height should be up to 4 m (13 ft) with a generous opening at the ridge up to 0.6 m (2 ft) suitably capped to prevent rain entry. A sharp angled pitch to the roof will help ventilation to be effective. There should also be an overhang on the roof beyond the eaves of up to 1 m (3 ft) to give protection from the heat of the midday sun. The curtains at the front or side should extend over 70–80% of the area and can, if desired, be controlled automatically by thermostats and motors with emergency 'fail-safe release' for high temperatures. Stocking rates for this type of building would be no more than about 7 broilers per m² (15 kg body weight per m²) or 4–5 layers or 3–4 breeders per m², depending on the size of the birds.

High air speeds are of great benefit to the birds and the attendants as they increase the heat loss by convection. Nevertheless it must be stressed that these speeds should be higher than are normal in poultry houses and there is some danger that if the temperature goes above 41 °C, which is the body temperature of the bird, high air speeds will *increase* the stress on the birds. Because of the importance of being able to increase the air movement whenever it is needed in naturally ventilated housing, it must be possible to open up as much as possible of the walls of the house without restriction. House design should allow for up to 100% opening of the sides in very warm areas. Careful thought must also be given to the siting of naturally ventilated buildings so the best use can be made of winds to flow through the house when required.

Controlled environment housing

This system is especially advocated for heavyweight broiler breeders or heavy broilers which cannot withstand very high temperatures because of their bulk and therefore poorer heat-dissipating abilities. It is also widely favoured for large cage laying houses where natural ventilation presents too many circulation difficulties. Stocking densities can be between 50 and 100% more than naturally ventilated housing and the principal features of controlled environment housing are as follows.

A high standard of thermal insulation is the first essential. The whole building should be insulated to a standard of 100 mm (4 in) polyurethane or the equivalent in other materials as chosen. Mechanical ventilation should be installed to a maximum of approximately double that in temperate climates. There is a general preference for positive pressure arrangements, as they enable a better control of air movement to be achieved and this is of especial importance in hot climates. In order to help the circulation of air it is also quite common practice to install ceiling circulating fans which may improve the environment in comparatively 'dead' areas with little air movement. Reliable electricity supplies and stand-by generators must be available.

It is noteworthy that building structures with a large thermal mass reduce the diurnal variation in temperature and in this way lower the extremes of environmental temperatures experienced by the birds. To put it simply, such buildings are slower to warm up in the day and to cool down in the night. In many parts of the world local materials are available which are ideal for this purpose, for example lightweight clay bricks or forms of aerated concrete. In buildings so constructed, the potentially large diurnal swings of temperature may also be further reduced by increasing the ventilation rate during the night and thereby cooling the whole structure of the house and then reducing the ventilation from its maximum in the heat of the day so that the building materials have a better opportunity to remain cool. It would be especially appropriate to use one of the water-cooling methods, described later, during the day to further assist the levelling out of temperature fluctuations. The temperature stresses that tend to kill poultry are caused largely by sudden rises in temperature, when the birds have had no chance to acclimatize; the method just described can be a significant help in preventing the most serious potentially lethal temperature stresses.

The main systems for keeping the birds cool use methods of evaporative cooling, of which there are four principal forms. The simplest is the *pad* or *filter* system in which the incoming air is drawn over a type of filter, often of a cellulose material, which is kept soaked in water. Provision has to be made to protect the pad from excessive sand or dust and recirculation and filtration of the water is also usually necessary.

A second system, also quite simple, is to use a series of *low pressure fogger nozzles* in the house, set up close to the ordinary fans or incoming air to assist in the distribution of the mist. This system tends to become quickly clogged and easily lends to uneven conditions with the litter near the fogger becoming dangerously damp.

There are two superior arrangements. The first is by the use of a *spinning disc* to generate a spray of small droplets which are passed into a stream of air. The most popular of the disc cooler systems comprise horizontal free-standing units. However a more recent development is the *ultra-high pressure mister* (Figure 2.15). In this case a pump is used to generate a high pressure in

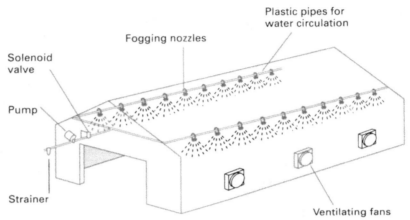

Figure 2.15 Illustration of a high-pressure misting evaporation cooling system in a poultry house.

reinforced plastic distribution tubes fitted with special nozzles. The small droplet particles pass out into the house at about 100 m/s (330 ft/s). The water supply must be carefully filtered and the pipes distributed in the house so that the incoming air will pick up the mist and help in the distribution.

The various cooling systems given here are capable of lowering the ambient temperature in the house by a maximum of about 10 °C (16 °F) when relative humidities are down to around 30%, but if the relative humidity is up to 50% the effect will be nearer 6 °C (10 °F) with a rise in relative humidity to 80%.

Poultry welfare and alternative systems

There is considerable world-wide concern about the possible inhumanity involved in some of the modern poultry production systems. The objections have arisen for two principal reasons—the restriction on the movement of birds that systems such as the battery cage impose, and the barren nature of the bird's surroundings, with birds spending their whole lives on a wire floor and restricted in movement by wire mesh or metal. Though considerable investigation is currently under way to try to establish the birds' mental and physiological reactions to environments such as the battery cage, results so far have given no definite answers. A satisfactory interim approach is epitomized in the attitude taken by the UK Farm Animal Welfare Council. The Council has suggested that much more attention should be given to the behavioural needs of the birds. All farm animals should be provided with the following:

1. Comfort and shelter;
2. Freedom from thirst, hunger or malnutrition;
3. Freedom of movement;
4. Prevention or rapid diagnosis and treatment of vice, injury and disease;
5. The company of other animals, particularly of like kind;
6. The opportunity to display most normal patterns of behaviour;
7. Adequate lighting;
8. Flooring which neither harms the animal nor causes undue strain;
9. The avoidance of unnecessary mutilation;
10. Emergency arrangements to cover fires and breakdowns.

The principal difficulty is with item 6, the opportunity to display most normal patterns of behaviour. For chickens this could well be said that the bird must be able to stand up, sit down, turn round, flap its wings, have dust baths and lay eggs in a bedded nest.

Because of the interest in satisfying these needs a number of 'alternative systems' to the battery cage and its barrenness and restriction have been researched and are also currently in use. The main systems which qualify for the description of 'alternative' are:

1. Free range
2. Straw-yard
3. Aviary and perchery
4. Deep litter
5. Modified cages, such as the 'get-away' cage

For the future it seems likely that interest in alternatives will concentrate on three major systems—*modified* free range, *covered* straw-yards, and *the aviary*—and these are described in the next paragraphs.

It is certain that the cost of producing laying eggs under any of the alternative systems will be greater than the cost of eggs produced from birds in cages. The consensus of opinion on the percentage extra cost of the alternatives compared with cage-produced eggs is shown in Table 2.2. The extra costs will be divided in a variable way according to the particular system used, but may include increased capital costs, extra costs on labour or feed, and additional

Table 2.2 Cost disadvantage of alternative egg production systems compared to battery cages

	Percentage increase in production costs over cages
Aviary, perchery and deep-litter	10–20
(Covered) straw-yard	20–30
(Traditional) free range	60–70
(Modified) free range	40–50

losses from mortality and broken or second quality eggs. It should be emphasized that the estimates given of extra costs are subject to considerable modification by skilful use of resources and by ingenuity in the maintenance of the environment and use of labour. In warmer countries the extra running costs may well be substantially reduced. It is encouraging to find that the costs of alternative systems are not prohibitive and the public is prepared to pay an extra amount so they can have their eggs produced in systems where birds have a more ethically acceptable environment.

The covered straw-yard

The straw-yard is basically a simple covered shed, uninsulated and naturally ventilated but giving good protection from the weather (Figure 2.16). An ideal structure is either an open-fronted monopitch house (lean-to) or simple pitched roof building. The floor must be deeply strawed—about 0.3 m (1 ft) deep and kept topped-up throughout the laying period. The birds are given a generous space of about 0.27 m² (3 ft²) each. The furniture of the house consists of nest boxes for laying (one box to five birds), hanging feeders and drinkers and movable perch units for roosting. Artificial lighting is provided to help boost winter egg production.

Our experience at Cambridge has been very satisfactory over a substantial period of time. The birds keep very active, spending a fair amount of time scratching in the straw, both searching for food and having dust baths.

Modified free-range system

Traditional free-range systems allow birds to roam freely over farmland at concentrations of up to 500 birds per hectare (200 birds per acre); the night roosting and egg nesting accommodation is simple and usually placed on sleds or wheels for regular movement. The problems of this system are so considerable and lead to such high costs of production that modified systems are now widely practised (Figure 2.17).

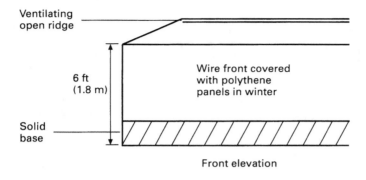

Ventilating open ridge

6 ft (1.8 m)

Wire front covered with polythene panels in winter

Solid base

Front elevation

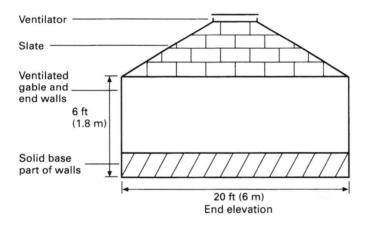

Ventilator

Slate

Ventilated gable and end walls

6 ft (1.8 m)

Solid base part of walls

20 ft (6 m)
End elevation

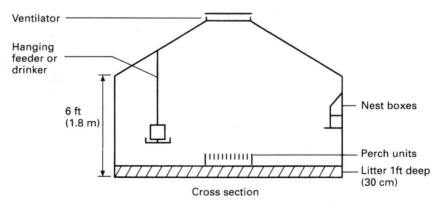

Ventilator

Hanging feeder or drinker

6 ft (1.8 m)

Nest boxes

Perch units

Litter 1ft deep (30 cm)

Cross section

Figure 2.16 Plans of covered straw-yard.

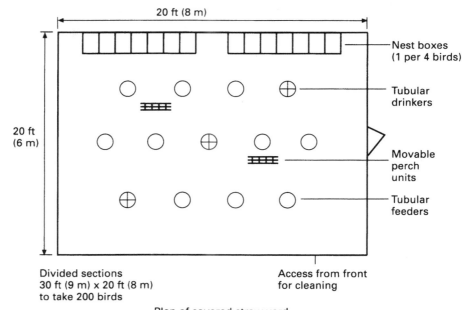

Plan of covered straw yard

Figure 2.16 Plans of covered straw-yard.

The housing should be thermally insulated and capable of containing the birds entirely during poor weather, for example deep snow, very hard frosts or in very wet conditions, all of which can be most harmful to the laying chicken. This housing may be permanent on a concrete base, or of a temporary type such as a semicircular polythene 'poly-pen' which can be moved from time to time. Electricity must be provided to give lighting to maintain winter egg production. Thus this part of the house is essentially a deep-litter or covered straw-yard.

An essential of the free-range system is that the birds must be able to go outside at all times during good weather and there should be palatable green-stuff for the birds to eat. Runs must be capable of being used in rotation and should be surrounded by fencing that is proof against predators, especially foxes. Birds must be shut up at night for safety and also to keep them warm.

It is highly dangerous to allow runs to become 'fowl sick' and once the pasture has been denuded it should be vacated, ploughed up and reseeded. If pasture is used carefully for birds, in a rotational programme, there will be several benefits. The good health of the birds will be assisted and the stocking density will be increased far above 500 birds per hectare in a particular run at any time; a factor of four times this will be acceptable and also of great benefit to the pasture before it is ploughed up.

It is probable that the use of modified free-range systems will have less

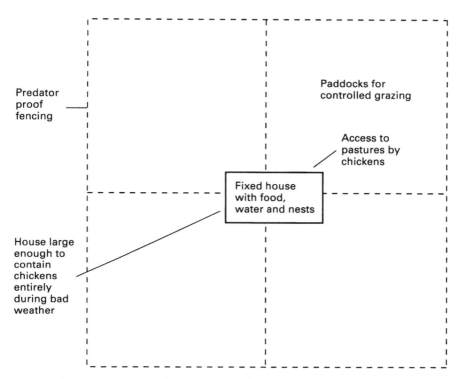

Figure 2.17 Plan of a modified free-range chicken unit.

application in temperate climates than in the warmer parts of the world. Credit is due to the pioneering farmers who are developing this arrangement by ingenious cost-saving methods. One farmer has recently built sheds with straw bales, using an internal aviary layout with multi-tiers of birds. With care this sort of housing may last as long as ten years with a very low capital input.

Aviary system for layers

Nearly ten years ago an aviary system was devised for broiler breeders on a farm in Hampshire which has subsequently been very thoroughly investigated and now is commercially used not only for breeders but also for layers. An aviary is essentially similar to a conventional deep-litter or slatted-floor system, but has the addition of extra floors of wire or slats. Feeders, drinkers and nest boxes are provided on each of the floors and the various levels are interconnected with ladders which are able to take both the birds and the attendants.

The great advantage of this system is that it allows the stocking density within the house to be much increased above that possible in an ordinary deep-litter or slatted-floor house. This reduces the capital cost per bird, enables a warmer house temperature to be maintained more akin to that in a cage laying house, and reduces feed consumption. Also, because of this extra warmth, ventilation may be increased thereby improving the litter conditions and generally eliminating condensation.

Aviary and perchery systems

A great deal of development has been expended on the development of aviaries and percheries. In essence these are controlled-environment houses with basically a deep-litter arrangement, but with the stocking density enormously increased by having either extra floors in the house—as in the aviary—or tiered perches as in the perchery. Birds have free access to all floors or tiers, they have feed and water at several levels and free access to nest boxes.

Birds in percheries may be stocked at 17–20 birds per m². The designs allow a high stocking density, enable good warmth to be maintained and appear to represent the most likely intensive development as an alternative to the cage system. Figure 2.18 shows the aviary system as developed at Gleadthorpe and now only generally used for breeders, while Figure 2.19 illustrates a type of perchery developed at Gleadthorpe and Figure 2.20 shows a second design evolved by Walter Michie at the West of Scotland College of Agriculture.

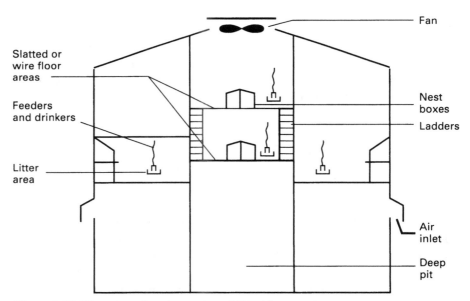

Figure 2.18 Diagrammatic cross-section of Gleadthorpe aviary.

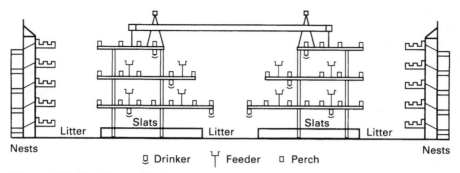

Litter   Slats   Litter   Slats   Litter

Nests   Nests

Drinker   Feeder   Perch

Figure 2.19 Gleadthorpe Perchery.

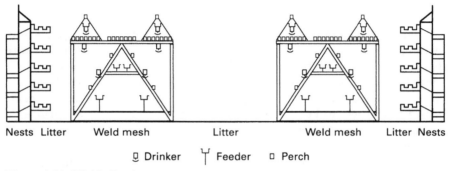

Nests Litter   Weld mesh   Litter   Weld mesh   Litter Nests

Drinker   Feeder   Perch

Figure 2.20 Michie Perchery.

Throughout all the trials with alternative systems in the UK and in other countries, it has been shown clearly that good management is far more crucial than with cage systems, together with the provision of a good environment, adequate space, the correct feeders, drinkers, perches and nests, appropriate stocking density and even the right breed of chicken and maintenance of good stocking rate.

Alternative systems for the future?

Research and investigation may eventually provide scientific answers to questions about welfare; meanwhile the moral issue has tended to make the running. Legislators, moved by public demand, may in future consider that keeping layers in multi-bird cages is unacceptable, in which case it is good to know that a number of alternative arrangements can be used to provide eggs of good quality, though at extra cost compared to those laid by the battery bird.

If the alternative systems to battery cages are to be successful in all respects, including welfare, the poultry farmer must be aware that good results will not come easily and management will require greater skills. Some of the most popular trends on which the modern poultry industry has been evolved will be abruptly halted or reversed and these must be considered in a practical manner.

Over several generations egg layers have been expertly bred for their efficiency under cage conditions and there will have to be certain charges in genetic selection techniques if the ideal strains for future needs are to be produced.

Diseases can be found to increase unless great care is taken. The birds can readily get infested with parasites and other disease agents in most alternative systems unless the litter is kept in a dry and friable state and only modest stocking rates are allowed. There will also be a revived risk of vices, such as feather pecking and cannibalism. It is unlikey that beak trimming will find acceptance, thus laying the onus entirely on skilled management as to whether vices are present or not.

Cages with their sloping wire bases almost certainly ensure the eggs are clean with no effort on the part of the attendant, but it can be very different with floor systems. If all the birds use the nest boxes provided, and if these are kept clean there is no problem, but quite unpredictably there may be a tendency for some or even a lot of birds to lay their eggs on the floor. This has many dangers. The eggs will probably be dirty and at the worst are even a danger to health. Some eggs may get broken and this may set in train 'egg-eating', which can cause a serious loss of eggs.

The final results depend on management. Just as the cage system has been the main factor which has encouraged the growth of the mammoth egg-laying units, so may the development of alternative systems see a change to smaller groups of birds in smaller buildings and on smaller poultry units. Many may applaud such a development. It will not only be an aid to good management but may also make better use of land resources. It is possible in the case of the smaller unit to utilize locally produced feedstuffs, and the litter at the end of the crop will be of great value to the land. If we can also see the removal of some of the hazards inherent in systems that are totally dependent on mechanical environmental control and feeding, there can be improved management since time is spent in the inspection of the birds rather than the repair of the machinery.

Further reading

Appleby M C, Hughes B O (1991) Welfare of laying hens in cages and alternative systems: environmental, physical and behavioural aspects. *World's Poultry Science Journal* 47: 109–28.

Austic R E, Nesheim M C (1990) *Poultry production.* Lea & Febiger, Ithaca, New York.

Clark J A (ed) (1981) *Environmental aspects of housing for animal production.* Butterworths, London.

Controlled environment for livestock (1990) Electricity Association Services, London.

Intensive livestock farming and animal protection (1990) Dutch Society for the Protection of Animals, The Hague.

Jordan F T W (ed) (1990) *Poultry diseases*, 3rd edn. Baillière Tindall, London.

Mead G C (ed) (1991) *Processing poultry.* Elsevier, Amsterdam.

Sainsbury D W B (1988) *Livestock health and housing.* Baillière Tindall, London.

THE HATCHERY AND HATCHING EGG

NIGEL E. HORROX BA, BVM&S, MRCVS

Introduction

Success in modern poultry production is very much dependent on being able to produce uniform, quality stock of a high health status. This, in turn, relies on quality management at the breeding and incubation stages of the production chain as this can greatly influence the quality of hatching eggs and the chicks they yield.

Good management also encourages good hygiene which will give returns on both the breeder farm and in the hatchery. This has a great influence on quality of both hatching eggs and chicks.

This chapter will concentrate on practices on the breeding farm and in the hatchery that, if correctly applied, should positively influence the quality and health status of the chicks the hatchery produces.

The egg

The first aspects to be considered are those of egg collection and transportation, but before discussing these two key areas of hatching egg management, consideration will be given to the egg. The egg contains a germinal disc that originated at fertilization from the genetic union of the male's spermatozoon and the female's ovum. This will develop into the chick. In addition, the egg contains all the nutrients, including the vitamins and minerals that the growing chick will require during incubation. The egg also contains large amounts of water. These reserves will also be drawn on for several days after hatching.

If deficiencies occurred in the breeder hen's diet these will be reflected in the eggs she produces and/or in their chicks.

This package of germinal disc and food supply for the developing chick is contained within the membranes and egg shell. These latter two play a key role in protecting the contents of the egg from external adversities. In embryonic development water and gaseous exchanges occur across the egg shell. Thus egg shell quality is very important because it has a role to play in maintaining an environment within the egg suitable for optimal embryonic development and in protecting the developing embryo from external adversities.

If the integrity of the shell is breached, for example by a micro-crack, the consequences are invariably catastrophic. A micro-crack will disturb the homeostatic balance to such an extent that so much water will be lost that the developing embryo will often die from dehydration. It will also provide an easy route by which microorganisms, for example spores of the fungus *Aspergillus*, can enter the egg.

Within the white of the egg are various substances that will counter microbial contaminants. The shell has on its outer surface a thin cuticle which, providing it remains intact, also plays an important role in the egg's defences.

Thus the fertile egg is not an item that can be abused at will—it is a highly complicated structure that must be handled carefully and be protected from external abuses of all kinds. This is just as important on the breeding farm as it is in the hatchery; as important when the egg is being stored as when the egg is being incubated.

Generally speaking, the egg is bacterially clean at the moment it is laid, although it may pick up some contamination as it leaves the cloaca. This can be particularly important in the spread of salmonella organisms, which will be considered later.

When the egg is laid it is at the bird's body temperature. Then it immediately starts to cool. During this cooling the contents of the egg shrink, but the shell, which is rigid, does not. This process sets up a pressure differential across the egg shell that causes air to be sucked into the egg through the numerous microscopic pores in the egg shell.

Nest-box management and egg collection

The key to successful egg handling on the farm is to minimize microbiological soiling of the egg when it is laid and throughout the period of cooling. To achieve this good nest-box hygiene is essential.

Several factors are important here. Firstly, nest-box contents should be kept clean and dry at all times. When they become dirty and/or damp they should be removed and replaced with fresh material. Secondly, the length of time the egg is in contact with nest-box material should be minimized. This is achieved by the regular collection of eggs at least three times a day. Some farms use roll-away nests that allow eggs to roll out of the nest after laying. This reduces the opportunity for soiling by the hens' feet. Thirdly, mixing a suitable solid disinfectant such as paraformaldehyde prills or flakes within the nest-box material may be considered. This approach must never be used as an alternative to good nest-box management and an adequate frequency of egg collection. However it can add a little bit of extra polish to on-farm egg handling.

Some farms now prefer nest-box pads made of Astroturf or a similar material. When these are used the same principles of nest-box management still apply. For reasons of hygiene, the best approach is to have 10–20% additional pads so that a soiled one can be removed and immediately replaced by a clean one while the soiled one is throughly cleaned, disinfected and dried.

The nest box is just the start when it comes to considering on-farm egg hygiene. From then, to the time the egg reaches the hatchery, anything that has contact with the egg may contaminate it. The manager must identify all these items and ensure all are kept as clean as is practically possible.

Such items include hands that have contact with the eggs, egg baskets, egg collecting trays and setter trays. To keep hands clean, adequate hand-washing facilities must be provided and staff must use them. Only paper towels should be used as cloth towels very quickly build up their own microbial burdens. A dirty cloth towel can quite easily replace a similar, or even a greater, number of microbes on the hands as those that have just been removed by washing.

Handling of eggs on the farm and during transportation to the hatchery is critical and they should be handled gently to avoid cracks or micro-cracks occurring. This is especially important with automatic egg collecting systems. Any point in the conveyor system at which eggs are jarred or forced against each other can result in the loss of a significant number of eggs, and hence chicks, over a year.

Egg hygiene

Nowadays, more and more hatching eggs are being washed on farm (Figure 3.1). This can be a very useful component in a total hygiene strategy—providing it is done correctly. Correct egg washing necessitates the use of a machine of the correct design: those utilizing a conveyor and wash sprays are prefer-

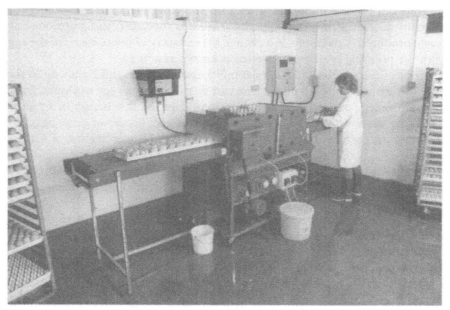

Figure 3.1 Egg washing and sanitizing machine used on a broiler breeder farm. (Photo courtesy of MS Technologies Ltd)

able. The farm manager must regularly check the egg washer to see that the chemicals are being used at the right concentrations and that the manufacturer's recommended temperature gradient for the various stages of the washing cycle is being adhered to.

Most egg washers work in two stages: firstly a washing stage with a detergent and then a sanitizing stage, usually with a chlorine compound.

Unfortunately no flock will lay all its eggs into the nest boxes. Some will be laid on the floor and these are known as 'floor eggs'. Traditionally 'floor eggs' were kept separate from nest eggs. The rationale behind this makes sense, but does it go far enough? Nowadays an approach of dividing eggs into clean and dirty eggs may be better. In other words a dirty nest-box egg has more in common with a traditional floor egg than does an egg laid on the floor in an area of clean litter!

Why is egg hygiene so important? It is because of what microbes can do to an egg. If bacteria get into the egg they find themselves in an ideal world with plenty of food and water; moreover, the egg shell also protects them from external adversities such as sunlight and disinfectants! Just for good measure the microbes are provided with the temperature they require for optimum growth as soon as the eggs are put into incubators!

When bacteria enter an egg they multiply rapidly. Very quickly one or two bacteria can become hundreds of millions and all of them are comsuming the contents of the egg, which is used by them as a foodstuff, and are producing waste products. This results in a change to the nature of the contents of the egg with the resulting egg becoming what is known as a 'rot'!

If one of the products of bacterial multiplication is gas this builds up in the egg. In time the build-up in pressure can be such that the egg explodes. Such eggs are called 'poppers', 'bangers' or 'exploders'. If this occurs in an incubator, the contents of this egg can be splattered over dozens of other eggs. As this material contains bacteria this can result in the contamination of further eggs.

Bangers are likely to explode whenever a tray of eggs is jarred as this can be just enough to tip the pressure differential to a point at which an explosion occurs.

In both 'rots' and 'bangers' embryonic death occurs and, if there are a significant number in a set of eggs, hatchability will be adversely affected.

However good egg hygiene is during egg collection, storage and incubation, some bacteria will survive. This is important as these will colonize the digestive tract of the newly hatched chicks and become their intestinal flora. This occurs much more slowly in eggs from incubated chicks than it does in naturally hatched ones.

If the egg shell is contaminated with pathogenic organisms these may enter the egg later in incubation or infect the chick at hatching or during the period while the chick remains in contact in the hatcher with shell debris and unhatched eggs. This causes infection in the young chick, which is usually seen as yolk sac infection. Chicks with yolk sac infection usually die up to 5 days of age. Antibiotic therapy is ineffective once the condition has started, but does help to lessen the bacterial challenge the chicks face.

Various factors influence the probability of these types of problems occurring. First and foremost, the egg or chick must come into contact with the problem-causing microorganisms. Spontaneous generation of microorganisms does not occur, so if good management keeps eggs and pathogenic bacteria apart, no problems will occur.

Good management will avoid egg contamination during production, collection, transportation, storage and incubation. In real terms this will never be totally achieved, so the aim must be to minimize contamination and to ensure that the egg is kept at all times in conditions that do not favour the multiplication of any bacteria that may already be on the egg shell. In particular, eggs should never be stored in an environment that induces condensation on the egg's surface as the moisture will make any dirt (microbial food) on the shell more rapidly available to the bacteria. Water is a prerequisite for rapid bacterial growth.

Temperature also has a similar effect. For this reason, eggs should be kept cool at 12 °C (55 °F) prior to incubation. In this context the management of on-farm and hatchery egg stores is important. Doors should not be left open; walls and ceilings should be well insulated and there should be no windows.

During this period temperatures should not fluctuate significantly as this can cause a stop/start phenomenon of the very early stage of embryonic development that can adversely affect hatchability.

Chick quality

The production of quality chicks necessitates that only quality eggs go into the incubators. Eggs that are too small or too large or double-yolked, eggs of abnormal shape or shell quality, damaged eggs and eggs showing excessive soiling should not be set.

Staff involved at each stage of the egg's passage from hen to hatchery have a quality control function to undertake in this context. None should assume that the responsibility for this exercise lies with another, although, obviously, the hatchery will have the final say as to which eggs are set.

There is a tendency in many large integrated companies to let standards of egg quality be eased when egg shortages occur in order that set numbers can be met. This has an impact on the uniformity and quality of the chicks produced. Thus if the decision to relax standards of egg grading prior to setting has to be taken it must be done by somebody who fully appreciates all the implications and ramifications of the decision to the company as a whole.

It may well be worth sacrificing chick numbers in order to maintain chick quality and, therefore, the productivity of the broiler and processing divisions of an integrator.

In view of the numbers of eggs involved in modern hatcheries precautions are taken at all stages of the cycle to counter bacterial growth. Egg washing has already been mentioned. In addition, eggs should be fumigated on farm or during transportation to the hatchery. During egg storage at the hatchery eggs should be regularly fogged with an appropriate product at least twice a week. Many hatcheries also subject eggs to a second fumigation prior to actual placement in the setters.

Incubation

Modern hatcheries tend to use multi-age setters, i.e. setters containing eggs of different ages. This practice means that a setter continually contains eggs, and staff will be regularly working in the setters. This will result in a build-up of the microbial load of the setter which is undesirable. This should be countered by fogging setters at least twice a week. Ideally this should be done after periods of activity in the machines.

The use of single-stage incubators has advantages when it comes to hygiene, but some would argue that these machines are not as efficient. If multi-stage machines are used, then a programme of closing machines down in turn so that they can be thoroughly stripped down, cleaned and disinfected should be adopted. Also as much cleaning as is practical should be undertaken before new eggs are put in the machine to replace those transferred to the hatchers.

During incubation the hatchery manager has a quandary—the conditions he or she needs to provide the egg in order to optimize hatchability and chick quality are also those that favour rapid microbial growth. For this reason, emphasis must be given to all aspects of hygiene management. Staff should never back-track in the hatchery, that is they should never go immediately from the take-off room to a setter. Work should flow from one end of the hatchery to the other (see Figure 3.2). Staff, especially in larger hatcheries, need to be disciplined in personal hygiene, designation of work areas and the use of specific clothing in specified areas.

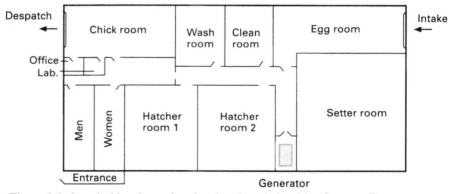

Figure 3.2 A typical hatchery plan showing the relationship of rooms. Eggs enter at one end, chicks are despatched from the opposite end. (Courtesy of B. Hodgetts, MAFF.)

Records

In today's hatcheries the use of detailed records is paramount as a means of quickly spotting a deviation from normal whatever the cause.

Every set of eggs should have its fertility and hatchability recorded by flock and machine. This enables a problem, should one occur, to be related as quickly as possible to a particular machine or flock. Other parameters that warrant recording are number of eggs rejected at grading (with reasons), the quality of the chicks produced and the liveability of the chicks in their first seven days of life. In addition, the incidence of any rots and bangers, culled chicks or dead-on-arrival chicks should be noted.

The amount of information involved here is large, but there are computer software packages that can greatly assist the recording and analysis of this information. There is no point in having the information if it is not regularly analysed. This should have the objective of quickly spotting areas of depressed performance. These recording systems need to interface with similar systems in the operations either side of the hatchery—the hatchery records must not be analysed in isolation. For example, it may be to the advantage of an integrator for a hatchery to be performing 5% below standard if both his breeding and fattening divisions are on or above standard.

In a similar fashion, it could be very expensive to have a hatchery performing to standard if this resulted in the breeding and fattening divisions failing to meet their standards. Of the total turnover of an agricultural division only a small percentage relates to the hatchery; often a small improvement in the fattening or breeding division is worth much more to the company than a larger improvement in the hatchery.

Thus, for example, at a company level a high standard of chick grading which reflects badly on the hatchery may be very beneficial to the concern as a whole as it gives a much greater return in the broiler operation and/or the processing plant.

Egg storage

With flocks performing differently and with differing numbers of chicks being required for placement, it is never possible to place all eggs in incubators the day they reach the hatchery. A situation known as egg banking thus occurs, in which the hatchery has to maintain a stock of eggs for setting. The effective management of this egg bank is essential. If egg age becomes too high (over 7–10 days for chickens) the performance of the eggs in the incubators is greatly depressed. One rule of thumb is that you can expect a 1% drop in hatchability for every day stored after a week of storage. This figure does vary between hatcheries.

Providing the egg bank does not become too large it can be used to advantage. For example, eggs from one breeder source can be bulked together to provide the chicks for a specified broiler, layer or turkey farm or sheds on it. Alternatively, the egg bank can give the hatchery enough flexibility so it can set eggs in sets according to age of breeder flocks of origin or egg weight bands.

The egg bank also has a key role in health management in that it can allow eggs from a known diseased flock to be segregated and hatched separately from others later in the day or on a designated day.

These attributes of the egg bank are only beneficial if the hatchery's records are good enough for it to know where all eggs are at all times. Also a policy on egg disposal should be defined that says eggs above a certain egg age, below a certain weight and above a certain weight are disposed of. With good planning and good management only the last two of these three should need to be used.

Hatchability problems

The incubation cycle is complex and will not be considered in detail here other than to say that successful incubation is very much dependent upon a combination of correct temperature, humidity, air flow, egg turning and hygiene during the incubation cycle. If any one of these parameters is not at its optimal level then the efficiency of the hatching process will be depressed. Sometimes this will just be reflected as chicks hatching off early or late; on other occasions it will show up as depressed hatchability or the production of poor quality chicks.

There are many causes of failure to hatch and the problems which can arise during incubation are considered in more detail in Appendix 3.1. The first problem which can be detected in the incubation cycle is lowered fertility. In hatchery terms percentage fertility is defined as the number of embryos still alive at test candling, which can be at 6–8 days of incubation for chicken eggs and 9–11 days for turkey eggs. A fertile egg is one in which fertilization has occurred.

The hatchery manager must be aware of this difference because although a poor test candling is often recorded as a poor fertility it may not be. In such instances eggs rejected at candling should be broken out and carefully examined. They should be categorized as clear, early dead or late dead. If the depressed fertility is due to an elevated number of clears then it is a true fertility problem.

The normal distribution (Figure 3.3) of clears, early deads and late deads is influenced by a whole host of factors including egg grading policy so the precise figures will vary between breeds, hatcheries, age of breeder flocks and management practices. For this reason the routine break-out of candling rejects from all flocks should be done so that the hatchery can establish its own data bank of normal values for clears, early deads and late deads.

When selecting eggs for candling, an adequate number of those set (usually

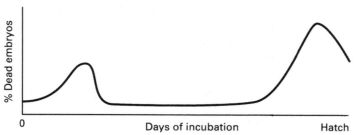

Figure 3.3 Curve showing normal embryonic mortality with the heaviest mortality occurring late in the incubation period.

1–5% depending on size of set) should be selected and the trays should reflect all machines and all positions in these machines. Data should be recorded by tray because if depressed fertility as defined by candling is found it may be because certain trays in certain incubators or all the trays in one incubator have distorted the reading. That is, the problem could be due to a machine or environmental fault and be nothing to do with the breeder flock or origin.

True infertility problems have their origins in a failure of fertilization. In the majority of instances this has its origins in a failure of mating on the farm. This could be because of lack of libido, an obesity problem or lameness in the cockerels. It could also be due to an inadequate number of cockerels.

If a true infertility has occurred then the first thing to do is to investigate the matter further at farm level. If the infertility is in reality due to an elevated early dead or late dead figure then its possible origins are many. These include nutrition, disease, turning failure, poor egg storage and incubator problems.

Depressed hatchability, which is considered to have occurred when more embryos than normal have died in the latter two-thirds of the incubation cycle, may be an entity in its own right or it may follow on from depressed fertility. The causes of depressed hatchability are many and are described in Appendix 3.1. They include egg age, nutrition, toxic factors, incubator management and disease.

'Rots' and 'bangers' already mentioned are the result of bacterial infection. In all cases the bacterial action causes odour and if there are only very few eggs affected in this way the experienced hatchery person will detect this 'off' smell in affected incubators.

Of the two, the banger is of more concern because when it explodes rotten egg material containing the causative bacteria is dispersed onto other eggs in the machine. They can then become infected and the whole situation can very quickly cascade out of control. The bacteria usually involved belong to the genus *Pseudomonas*. Pseudomonads vary in their ability to produce gases, and different organisms impart different colours to the rotten egg material, ranging from purple to blue and green to black and grey.

This type of problem tends to exhibit two different epidemiological patterns. In the first, the incidence of affected eggs is low and an investigation usually reveals a distinct pattern, be it in eggs from young flocks, eggs from flocks with floor egg problems, eggs that have been excessively buffed (hand cleaned) or just eggs from certain farms. In these instances the contamination has arisen on farm and a careful analysis of the problem will highlight areas in which management attention should reduce or even eliminate the problem.

The other pattern seen is one in which the number of affected eggs suddenly increases dramatically. This picture is usually associated with a malfunction of an egg washer or dipping equipment (see later). In both instances the malfunction has resulted in the eggs being washed or dipped in a bacterial soup. Alternatively, problems in temperature control mean the egg is cooling at a time when it should not be and this causes bacteria to be sucked into the centre of the egg via its pores.

Another microbial entity that causes losses in the incubation cycle is the one commonly called fungal air-cell. In this condition embryonic death occurs associated with a massive fungal growth in the egg's air-cell. *Aspergillus* species are the fungi usually involved. The word 'associated' is used deliberately as there is considerable debate as to whether the fungal growth causes the embryonic death or whether it is coincidental. This is because many eggs showing this condition have enlarged air-cells due to water loss from the egg, which is in itself fatal to embryos. A common cause for this is micro-cracks and these also provide an easy route of entry for fungal spores.

When fungal air-cell problems involve more than the occasional egg (incidences can be as high as 8–12%) the problem disappears when measures are instituted to eliminate the occurrence of micro-cracks.

Yolk sac infection

If the various management factors described fail, chicks may hatch and develop yolk sac infection (Plate 4). This can arise for the following reasons:

1. Contaminated eggs from the breeder farm;
2. Failure to control humidity or temperature in the incubator;
3. Infection from the environment within the hatchery;
4. Failure to control temperature in the chick holding area.

Yolk requires energy from the chick to resorb into the body, so that any condition which devitalizes the tissues prevents this and makes conditions more suitable for infection. Thus incorrect humidity or temperature control delays the withdrawal of yolk into the abdominal cavity. Any remnants of yolk sac tissue protruding from the navel are more susceptible to infection. Bacteria multiply in the yolk producing toxins which causes death in 3–4 days.

Disease prevention strategies

In modern poultry production the hatchery is the link between the breeding operation and the production (meat or table eggs) operation. It is, therefore, imperative that management institutes procedures that ensure that the hatchery and its vehicles do not backtrack infections from the production to the breeding operation or spread disease between the farms.

For this reason, a policy of segregating staff into those who deal with the eggs on receipt and early in incubation and those who work in the hatcher rooms and handle chicks, should be adopted. There should be no cross-over of staff. In a similar vein, vehicles collecting eggs from the breeder farms and those delivering chicks to their recipient farms should only be used for their designated role and they should not do each other's jobs. Also the egg receiving station should be as far away as possible from the chick despatch point. These should preferably be on opposite sides of the hatchery building.

In the design of a hatchery, consideration should be given to air flow: air should always move in the same direction as the product flows through the hatchery. It is also important that exhaust air from the hatchers is not expelled at a point close to where air is drawn for use in the setters. Better still, all incoming air should pass through microbial filters and positive air pressure should be used to ensure air does not flow inside the hatchery from dirty to clean areas.

The hatchery is the hub to the whole operation and management procedures should be in place to protect it. As an instance, all incoming eggs should be examined upon receipt and unsatisfactory loads, such as ones with a high incidence of dirty eggs, should be rejected.

Hatchery hygiene

General hygiene in the hatchery is critical because the possibility of cross-over contamination in the hatchery is a real one. For example, only one shed of breeder layers may be salmonella positive, but slack management procedures and poor hygiene at the hatchery could mean that the vast majority of chicks being produced by that hatchery are contaminated by salmonella.

Security of inputs is therefore critical. All eggs should be fumigated on the vehicle before arrival or before setting. Here management has a key role to ensure that this procedure is always undertaken and that it is effective.

Where a fumigation cabinet is used, factors like poor circulation of fumigant, solid sides to trolleys, leaks from the cabinet, porous materials within the cabinet that absorb fumigant and surface water that acts in a similar way are all critical. The effectiveness of fumigation cabinets should be regularly evaluated.

Eggs are not the only input into a hatchery that can introduce a problem. Staff are also very important. If the hatchery is of a reasonable size it is sensible to insist that all staff shower in and then only wear clothing provided by the company that remains on site. Staff should not take any foodstuff into a work area—it is best if foodstuffs are confined to a canteen area.

Humans like any other animals can harbour salmonella organisms so, in larger hatcheries, a stool testing programme for staff is quite justifiable. If this is not done there should at least be a procedure whereby staff report any sickness and diarrhoea to management. This procedure is especially pertinent in countries where the isolation of certain salmonella serotypes from breeding or table egg flocks can result in that flock's statutory slaughter.

In addition to this a thorough and regular cleaning and disinfection programme is essential. All areas should be thoroughly cleaned and disinfected after use and areas that are in continual use, such as egg stores, corridors and canteen facilities, should be treated in a similar fashion each week. The cleaning programme should not overlook areas like the changing rooms, office, sleep areas or external concrete surrounds. In these two areas the manager has key responsibilities. Firstly, he or she should be aware of everything that enters the hatchery and have in place a procedure for minimizing the risk that it presents. These risks may be anything from an engineer who undertakes some key repair work to a delivery of new brushes and mops.

Hygiene monitoring

The good manager will regularly test the effectiveness of his cleaning programme and the cleaners who implement it. In this instance he will take samples for laboratory testing. Here it should be remembered that microbiological testing of the effectiveness of cleaning is a management tool and not a scientific exercise.

Thus it is far better to test 50 areas and be told which are clean and which are dirty than to test 10 areas and obtain a highly accurate bacterial count from each. It does not matter to the hatchery manager whether a surface has 1.02 or 1.03 million bacteria per square centimetre as they are both dirty! In practice both these testing regimes would cost about the same, so it is far better to test 50 areas.

However, having undertaken the test and received the results, the manager must ensure that they are used properly. Results from hygiene tests should be used to motivate staff—it is just as important, if not more so, to show staff good results and praise them, than to show them bad results and scold them. Only a bad manager shows staff the bad results alone.

Once staff have been made aware of areas that did not score well on the hygiene test, the next test should be used to check that staff are now cleaning those areas properly. It is also important to ensure that the areas tested, and the day on which the test is undertaken, vary as staff should not be able to concentrate their efforts on the areas they know are going to be tested!

The manager should utilize his hygiene reports to spot trends that can help the job of management. This is best done using a graphical approach that visually represents improvements, deteriorations or seasonal trends.

Hatching

At the end of the incubation period the chicks hatch. This period and the one immediately after it are critical for the production of good chicks. It should be emphasized, though, that hatching and chick handling cannot make bad chicks good but can certainly make good chicks bad!

Ideally all the chicks should hatch over a short a period as possible. If the period is extended or if hatching occurs earlier or later than it should, there is a fault in the incubators and it is most likely to be related to temperature or humidity levels.

A hatch is ready to pull when 95–97% of the hatchlings are dry, i.e. when 3–5% show evidence of some wet down. If they are all dry, then pulling is late and the chicks may have suffered from dehydration. If most are still damp they should be allowed to stay in the hatcher a little longer so that post-pull chilling is avoided.

Many hatcheries still place some formalin in the hatchers as the last stage of their hygiene programme. If chicks are pulled gasping or with a rattling sound in their windpipes it is likely that they have been exposed to excessive formalin gas by this procedure.

Grading, sexing and vaccination

After pulling, the hatchlings go through a series of activities—some or all of grading, sexing, toe trimming, desnooding in the case of poults, beak tipping, spray vaccination, vaccination by injection, administration of antibiotics by injection and boxing. All of this can be stressful so the hatchery manager and the staff must ensure that all these tasks are done quickly and efficiently with as little stress as possible being imposed on the hatchlings. There should also be a periodic review to see if all the procedures currently being undertaken still need to be done—it is surprising how many hatcheries perform certain tasks simply because they have always done them!

Some of these activities will now be considered in more detail. Grading is a very subjective exercise so that the base level for downgrades can only be determined by the hatchery. At grading, signs that are indicative of problems elsewhere should be looked for. If most of the downgrading is for unhealed navels, problems with the incubators, especially in relation to humidity, are worthy of further investigation.

Sexing is usually done by feather sexing (Figure 3.4) although occasionally, and especially in turkeys, it is done by vent sexing. Both grading and sexing require handling. If this is rough, mortality can ensue. This can be checked by taking dead in-box chicks and first-day dead chicks from the farm for a post-mortem examination. In some hatcheries there are systems for automatically marking the chicks handled by each member of staff using different colours of inks. Then, if sexing and grading damage is detected at a check post-mortem examination, the proportion of damage attributable to each member of staff can be ascertained.

Toe trimming, desnooding and beak tipping should only be undertaken by mature, competent, well-trained staff and management should routinely evaluate each operator's standard of workmanship. This is done by taking 100 chicks that the operator has processed and carefully examining and recording their work standards. In cases of unacceptable work, additional training should be given or the operator should be allocated to a different task.

When vaccination is being undertaken it is critical that every chick receives its required dose. This is critical for injected vaccines, but not so important for some of the spray vaccines such as infectious bronchitis H120, as in this instance the vaccinal virus, can circulate amongst chicks in the period after vaccination.

When live vaccines are being given it must be stressed that they are indeed live and can be killed. This can inadvertently happen by using disinfectant on the vaccinating or mixing equipment. Such vaccines should be stored according to the manufacturers instructions so that none of their potency is lost.

In the case of either dead or live vaccines that are administered by injection it is essential that every bird receives its dose. This can be checked by incorporating a harmless dye into one batch of vaccine and then examining chicks post-vaccination to ensure they have actually received their dose.

In some countries chicks or poults are given an antibiotic injection at the hatchery. This practice should only be used as part of a control programme for

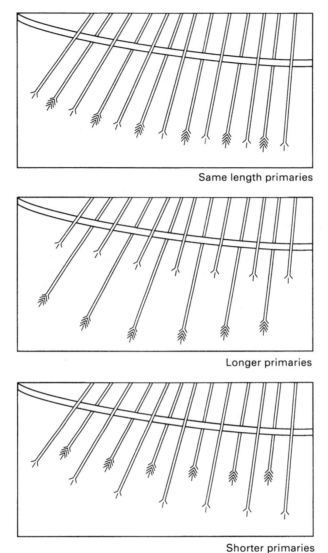

Same length primaries

Longer primaries

Shorter primaries

Figure 3.4 Feather sexing of broilers is possible by observing the relationship between the coverts (upper layer) and the primaries (lower layer) on the outer half of the wing.

diseases like arizonosis—it should never be adopted as a substitute for good management and high standards of hygiene. In addition to vaccination, some hatcheries now administer a competitive exclusion product as part of their salmonella avoidance programme.

Record keeping

Records are the key to successful management in the hatchery. Some examples of their use have already been mentioned. In some of the newer hatcheries it is now possible to centralize all recording into a computer. This can include the regular monitoring for parameters such as temperature, humidity, turning and alarms that all incubators are recording continually.

Thus, with the correct computer program, it should be possible to relate the performance of broilers on the ground to the hatch data, which in turn can be related to the incubators the eggs were in and the breeder flocks that supplied the eggs. So performance can now be analysed in great detail, but, here again, this information is only of value if management is prepared to use it to make future production even more efficient.

In addition to records, how can the manager pinpoint a problem? Candling has previously been mentioned as has the use of the break-out technique to evaluate true fertility. Egg break-out is used to examine dead in-tray eggs to determine the reasons for failure of the eggs to hatch. Appendix 3.1 shows the principal causes of failure to hatch with some of the corrective measures required. Examination of dead-in-shell should be carried out at least weekly for every flock using a chart to record the results (Figure 3.5).

* Embryo examination

Flock number..   Date..,...

Infertile	Early	Middle	Late	Malposition	Freaks	Rotten / bangers
	Day 0–5	Day 6–18	Day 19–21			

* Examine 25 dead-in-shell eggs per flock.

Figure 3.5 Chart for recording dead-in-shell examinations.

It can be very difficult after 21 days of incubation to tell the difference between an early dead germ and an infertile egg, as a certain amount of deterioration of the egg contents will have occurred. With experience the hatchery manager can undertake a meaningful break-out analysis. With practice he or she should be able to accurately age dead embryos and to pick up tell-tale signs such as clubbed down, ectopic viscera, additional limbs and subcutaneous haemorrhaging. These data can then be interpreted by the manager or his advisers.

As the manager builds up a database of information derived from this kind of exercise he will be able to define acceptance limits for certain parameters and know how these are influenced by factors such as age of breeder flock of origin, egg age and incubator characteristics.

In addition to checks on the eggs, checks can be undertaken on the environment the eggs are first stored in and then incubated in. In the smaller hatcheries these may still be done manually, but in the larger ones they will be recorded automatically on paper charts or by computer. Here again the hatchery manager will be able to build up a database, which will help define which environmental pattern produces the best results for eggs of differing types— breed, breeder flock or egg age. His end goal may be total hatchability or hatchability expressed as grade 1 hatchlings or hatchability related to seven-day liveability figure.

Whichever yardstick is used it will, in time, be possible to define which sequence of environmental happenings in the incubation cycle give the best results. Once this has been defined it should be possible to define how much performance varies according to variations in particular parameters, for example for each additional day of egg storage.

Salmonella

The importance of the salmonella bacterium has increased dramatically in recent years since it assumed a political role to complement its pathogenic one. The role of salmonella must be put into context. Only a few serotypes out of some 3000 cause disease in poultry. The vast majority of serotypes, when they happen to be present in poultry, do not cause any adverse effect on the bird— they lie dormant in its digestive tract.

However, techniques at the processing plant can result in carcase or meat contamination of product. This, in itself, may not be of too much concern. What is of concern is if that product is abused then low numbers of salmonella organisms can multiply up to a level at which they are capable of causing food poisoning in man. Most salmonella serotypes, given the right set of circumstances, can cause food poisoning.

Nowadays the responsible poultry producer will be doing everything possible to stop salmonella organisms entering the production chain. Within this the hatchery has a key role to play. Firstly, the hatchery manager needs to ensure that salmonella organisms are not introduced into the production chain at the hatchery level. Secondly, in the event that a salmonella organism is already present, for example in one breeder flock, the hatchery manager must ensure that practices at the hatchery do not greatly increase the numbers of salmonellae nor do they allow the organisms to back-track to other breeder flocks. The former requires the manager to define all the possible routes by which salmonella could enter the hatchery and then institute management practices to counter these risks. Aspects of hatchery management relevant to the risk of infection back-tracking have already been considered in this chapter.

Conclusion

Modern hatchery management is not just about eggs. It is also about systems management and people management and to be successful today's hatchery manager has to blend all of these together. In addition modern hatchery management is also about spotting deviations from normal as early as possible and rectifying them as quickly as possible. The importance of efficient, effective record keeping in this can not be underestimated.

Further reading

Solomon S E (1991) *Egg and eggshell quality.* Iowa State University Press (USA), Wolfe Publishing (outside USA). London.
Tullett S G (1991) *Avian incubation. Poultry Science Symposium No. 22.* Butterworth-Heinemann, London.

Appendix 3.1

Examination of dead in shell to determine cause of embryo mortality

Problem	Probable causes	Suggested corrective measures
1. Eggs clear—no blood rings, no embryonic development.	A. Eggs infertile due to:	A. Proper breeding, nutrition and flock management practices.
	i. Too many or too few males. Males fighting or interfering with each other.	i. Follow recommendations of your breeder.

Problem	Probable causes	Suggested corrective measures
	ii. Males too old.	ii. Do not use old males unless proved valuable breeders.
	iii. Inadequate nutrition or insufficient water (or water too warm/too cold).	iii. Check ration and water distribution.
	iv. Birds too crowded.	iv. Provide adequate space per bird in housing.
	v. Wet litter causing foot lesions in males.	v. Provide comfortable housing with dry litter ensuring adequate ventilation. Level of water in drinkers should be carefully controlled.
	vi. Disease in the flock.	vi. Carry out approved disease control practices.
	vii. Males overweight.	vii. Control bodyweight to breeder's recommendation.
	B. Eggs damaged either by being badly chilled or overheated.	B. Gather eggs often, cool properly and quickly.
	C. Eggs held to long, or held under improper conditions of temperature and humidity.	C. Eggs kept under proper temperature and humidity conditions and set within 10 days after date laid.
	D. Improper fumigation.	D. Do not fumigate eggs in the first stages of incubation.
2. Eggs candling clear—but showing blood ring or very small embryo on breaking.	A. Badly chilled eggs or eggs overheated or held at too high a temperature.	A. Protect eggs against freezing temperatures, gather eggs often, cool properly and quickly, hold eggs under conditions recommended by breeder.
	B. Improper incubator temperature at earliest stage of incubation.	B. Check accuracy of thermometer. Operate incubator at proper temperature.

Problem	Probable causes	Suggested corrective measures
	C. Improper fumigation— too much fumigant, fumigant not cleared from machine soon enough, or eggs fumigated too early in the incubation period.	C. Do not fumigate between the 12th and 96th hours of incubation. In any fumigation of eggs, use approved procedures and quantities. Prefumigation before placement in the incubator is preferable to fumigation of eggs in the incubator.
	D. Breeding flock out of condition or disease.	D. Do not set eggs from diseased birds, particularly those infected with pullorum or other salmonella diseases.
	E. Improper nutrition of flock.	E. Feed properly balanced ration of high quality.
	F. Eggs held too long, or held under improper conditions of temperature and humidity.	F. Keep eggs under proper temperature and humidity conditions and set within 10 days after date laid.
	G. Embryos infected with organisms from dams, or, especially, by external microbial contamination through shell.	G. Concentrate on good egg hygiene practices.
3. Many dead germs (1st to 6th days of incubation).	A. Temperature too high or too low in incubator.	A. Check accuracy of thermometer. Operate incubator at proper temperature.
	B. Lack of ventilation.	B. Provide adequate ventilation of the incubator room and proper openings of the incubator ventilators. Do not re-circulate foul air. Supply 100% fresh, tempered air.
	C. Improper turning of eggs.	C. Turn eggs hourly, or at least at regular intervals eight times daily.

Problem	Probable causes	Suggested corrective measures
	D. See probable causes C, D, E, F & G in problem 2 above.	D. See suggested corrective measures C, D, E, F & G in problem 2 above.
4. Any considerable number of embryos dead from the 6th through the 16th days incubation (normally this is a period of relatively low embryonic death).	A. Incubator temperature much too high.	A. Check accuracy of thermometer. Operate incubator at proper temperature.
	B. Infected embryos— either by infection from dams, or especially by external microbial contamination through shell.	B. Concentrate on good egg hygiene practices.
	C. Lack of ventilation.	C. Provide adequate ventilation of the incubator room and proper openings of the incubator ventilators.
	D. Improper nutrition of the flock, especially vitamin deficiency.	D. Feed properly balanced ration of high quality.
5. Chicks fully formed, but dead without pipping. May have considerable quantities of unabsorbed yolk (18 to 21 days of incubation).	A. Low average humidity in incubator; humidity too low or too high at transfer time in hatcher.	A. Maintain proper humidity throughout incubation and hatching cycle.
	B. See probable causes A, B & C in problem 3 above.	B. See suggested corrective measures A, B & C for problem 3 above.
	C. Temperature too low or too high (more probably too high) in hatcher.	C. Check accuracy of hatcher thermometer. Operate at proper temperature.
	D. Lack of ventilation in hatcher.	D. Provide adequate ventilation of the hatcher room and proper openings of the hatcher ventilators.
	E. Chilled eggs.	E. Gather eggs quickly, cool properly and hold under proper conditions.
	F. Infected embryos.	F. See 2G.
	G. Disease or flock in poor condition.	G. Diagnosis and correct flock factors.

Problem	Probable causes	Suggested corrective measures
6. Eggs pipped, but chicks dead in shell. (Hole made in shell but embryo failed to pip further. Embryo may still be alive.)	A. Low average humidity.	A. Maintain proper humidity levels throughout incubation and hatching cycle.
	B. Inadequate ventilation or excessive fumigation during course of hatch.	B. Provide adequate ventilation of the incubator room and proper openings of the incubator ventilators. Follow approved methods with regard to fumigation in the hatcher. Do not re-circulate foul air. Supply 100% fresh, tempered air.
	C. Excessive high temperature for a short period.	C. Guard against temperature surge.
	D. Low average temperature.	D. Maintain proper temperature throughout incubation and hatching cycle.
	E. Infected embryos.	E. See 2G. Check hatcher sanitation procedures. Make sure hatcher and hatch trays have been thoroughly cleaned, disinfected and fumigated after each hatch. Properly fumigate in hatcher after transfer.
7. Eggs pipped part way, embryos either dead or still alive.	A. Eggs set large end down in incubator trays or, less likely, crowded in hatcher trays so that some eggs are large end down.	A. Check egg setting and transfer procedures and be certain eggs are set and transferred properly.
	B. Improper turning of eggs.	B. Turn eggs hourly, or at least at regular intervals eight times daily.
	C. Low average humidity.	C. Maintain proper humidity levels throughout the incubation and hatching cycle.

Problem	Probable causes	Suggested corrective measures
	D. Inadequate ventilation, excessive fumigation during course of hatch, or chicks weakened from other causes.	D. Provide proper ventilation of the incubator and hatcher rooms and proper openings of the incubator and hatcher ventilators. Do not re-circulate foul air. Follow approved methods with regard to fumigation in the hatcher. Investigate for disease and contamination and check all aspects of flock management, egg handling and egg storage (see problem 6E above).
	E. Excessive high temperature.	E. Guard against temperature surge.
	F. Low average temperature for a short period.	F. Maintain proper temperature throughout incubation and hatching cycle.
8. Sticky chicks—chicks smeared with egg contents.	A. Low average temperature.	A. Use proper operating temperature.
	B. Average humidity too low.	B. Maintain proper humidity levels throughout incubation and hatching cycle.
	C. Inadequate ventilation or improper fumigation of eggs in incubator, or excessive fumigation in the hatcher.	C. Provide adequate ventilation of the incubator room and proper openings of the incubator ventilators. Follow approved methods with regards to fumigation. Do not re-circulate foul air. Supply 100% fresh, tempered air.

Problem	Probable causes	Suggested corrective measures
9. Shell sticking to chicks.	A. Eggs dried out.	A. Maintain proper humidity levels during egg-holding period and throughout incubation and hatching cycle. Do not over-ventilate.
	B. Low humidity at hatching time.	B. Proper humidity levels throughout incubation and hatching cycle.
	C. Improper egg turning.	C. Turn eggs hourly, at regular intervals eight times daily.
10. Chicks hatching too early with bloody navels.	A. Temperature too high.	A. Maintain proper temperature levels throughout incubating and hatching cycle.
11. Rough, congested or poorly healed navels.	A. High temperature or wide temperature variations.	A. Maintain proper temperature levels throughout incubation and hatching cycle.
	B. Excessive humidity in hatcher after transfer.	B. Use less humidity during first 24–36 hours after transfer.
	C. Embryos infected prior to transfer or during hatching.	C. See 2G and 6E.
12. Chicks too small.	A. Small eggs.	A. Usually 50 g standard minimum size.
	B. Low humidity during egg holding and/or incubation.	B. Maintain proper humidity levels during egg-holding period and throughout incubation and hatching cycle.
	C. High temperature.	C. Maintain proper temperature throughout incubation and hatching cycle.
13. Large, soft-bodied, mushy chicks— chicks dead on trays with bad odour.	A. Low average temperature.	A. Maintain proper temperature throughout incubation and hatching cycle.

Problem	Probable causes	Suggested corrective measures
	B. Poor ventilation in incubator and/or hatcher.	B. Provide proper ventilation of the incubator and hatcher rooms and proper openings of the incubator and hatching ventilators.
	C. Humidity too high, especially during incubation.	C. Maintain proper humidity levels throughout incubating and hatching cycle.
	D. Omphalitis (navel infection).	D. Fumigate eggs before setting in incubator. Thoroughly clean and fumigate hatcher and hatch trays between hatches. Fumigation is useless if trays are soiled with organic matter. Be sure hatch trays are clean.
14. Weak chicks.	A. Excessive temperature in hatcher.	A. Do not permit temperature in hatcher to be too high. If chicks are to be held in hatcher, reduce temperature after hatch completed.
	B. Inadequate ventilation in hatcher.	B. Provide adequate hatcher room ventilation. Maintain adequate ventilator openings in hatcher. Open ventilators wider as hatch progresses. Properly remove hatcher exhaust air. Do not re-circulate.
	C. Excessive fumigation in hatcher at hatching time.	C. Follow approved fumigation practices.
	D. Disease, poor nutrition or flocks otherwise in poor condition.	D. Diagnose and correct flock factors.
	E. Infected embryos.	E. See 2G and 6E.

Problem	Probable causes	Suggested corrective measures
15. Short down on chicks or eyes stuck closed with down.	A. High temperature.	A. Maintain proper temperature levels throughout incubating and hatching cycle.
	B. Low humidity.	B. Maintain proper humidity levels throughout incubating and hatching cycle.
	C. Excessive ventilation in hatcher at hatching time.	C. Reduce openings of hatcher ventilators. Do not restrict so far as to permit animal heat to build temperature above safe level.
	D. Holding chicks in hatcher too long after hatch.	D. Remove as soon as chicks are fluffed and ready.
16. Delayed hatch— eggs not starting to pip until 21st day or later.	A. Average temperature too low, especially in the hatcher.	A. Maintain correct temperature levels throughout incubation and hatching cycle.
	B. Eggs held too long.	B. Try not to hold eggs more than 7 to 10 days, 14 days at most, and then only if holding conditions ideal.
	C. Weakened, infected embryos.	C. See 2G and 6E.
	D. Delayed hatch of large eggs or old eggs when mixed with smaller or fresher eggs.	D. Where possible, try to set eggs of uniform size and age per machine. Larger eggs or eggs which have been held longer frequently give better hatching results when incubated at slightly higher temperature than for smaller or fresher eggs. Alternatively, set larger or older eggs a few hours earlier than smaller or fresher eggs so that development will be roughly equal at transfer.

Problem	Probable causes	Suggested corrective measures
17. Prolonged hatch—some chicks early, but hatch slow in finishing. (Frequently associated with 19, 20 or 21-day embryos still in the shell with excessive unabsorbed yolk sac. All yolk must be absorbed by end of 20th day.)	A. Improper gathering, cooling and holding of eggs.	A. Eggs must be gathered frequently, cooled properly before boxing and held at proper temperature and humidity before setting.
	B. Mixing large eggs and small eggs in the same setting. (Large eggs are usually from older hens or heavier breeders, small eggs from younger hens or lighter breeders. Larger eggs and older eggs tend to hatch later than small eggs, all other things being equal.)	B. See 16D.
	C. Hot spots and cold spots due to (1) improper incubation design, or (2) using cooling water that is excessively cold, or (3) supplying the incubator with air under too much pressure or air which has not been pre-conditioned or (4) pumping exhaust air out of the machine in a manner which interferes with the machine's own circulation system.	C. Consult incubator manufacturer for correct operation.
	D. Improper incubator or hatcher temperature.	D. Maintain proper temperature levels throughout incubating and hatching cycle.
	E. Re-circulating stale, contaminated air.	E. Ventilate properly, with 100% fresh, tempered air.

Problem	Probable causes	Suggested corrective measures
18. Malformed chicks in poor hatch, usually associated with an excessive number of chicks dead in the shell with a high incidence of malpositions.	A. Eggs held too long before setting, even under good conditions, or eggs held any length of time at improper levels of temperature and/or humidity.	A. Try not to hold eggs more than 10 days if at all possible, and then only if holding conditions ideal.
	B. Eggs chilled before setting.	B. Gather eggs quickly, cool properly before boxing and hold under proper conditions.
	C. Improper turning or setting.	C. Set eggs small end down only, in the incubator. Turn eggs hourly, or at least at regular intervals 8 times daily. Be sure you do not trap eggs large end down on transfer.
	D. Inadequate ventilation.	D. Provide adequate ventilation of the incubator and hatcher room and proper openings of the incubator and hatcher ventilators. Do not re-circulate foul air. Supply 10% fresh, tempered air.
	E. Abnormally high or abnormally low incubator temperature.	E. Maintain proper temperature levels throughout the incubation and hatching cycle.
	F. Insufficient moisture.	F. Maintain proper humidity levels throughout the incubation and hatching cycle.
	G. Flock diseases or egg contamination.	G. See 2G.

Problem	Probable causes	Suggested corrective measures
	H. Improper nutrition or use of feed which has been mixed with inappropriate drugs or with fungicide or other poisons.	H. Use properly balanced breeder feed of high quality, made with grain which has not been treated with fungicides or other chemicals.
	I. Damage to eggs in shipment caused by jarring or shipping large end down.	I. Hatching eggs must be shipped in good quality, well-protected egg cases, or equivalent, with small end down. Avoid rough handling.
19. Special cases of crippled and malformed chicks.		
A. General with regard to all malformations.	A. Disease, contamination, toxic feed or improper nutrition must always be suspected whenever crippled or malformed chicks are encountered.	A. See 2G.
B. Crooked toes.	B. Improper temperature. This can also be caused by setting too few eggs per tray, permitting too much freedom of movement to chicks too soon.	B. Maintain proper temperature levels throughout incubating and hatching cycle. Do not set too few eggs per tray.
C. Spraddle legs.	C. Caused by hatching trays which are too smooth.	C. Use crinoline cloth or rough creped paper in hatch trays.
D. Cross beak, twisted beak, etc.	D. Heredity (lethal genes).	D. Not usually necessary.
20. Exploders— problem usually occurs at about 12–13 days of incubation.	A. Badly contaminated floor eggs.	A. See 2G and 6F.

Problem	Probable causes	Suggested corrective measures
	B. Improper washing of eggs, or wiping or buffing eggs with contaminated equipment.	B. If eggs are washed, use only approved equipment, detergents and solutions at adequate temperature. Renew solutions before they become contaminated. Do not, under any circumstances, use washing solutions below (or above) recommended temperatures.
	C. 'Sweating' of eggs after removal from cooler.	C. Hold eggs at approved temperatures, neither too high, nor too low.
	D. Fogging of eggs in incubator or other splattering eggs with water.	D. Improper cleaning or adjustment of the humidifying mechanism can cause water to be thrown on the eggs, so appropriate maintenance instructions should be followed.
	E. Contamination from previous exploders. This is a problem which multiplies rapidly unless stopped.	E. The best means of control of exploders is to prevent them occurring in the first place. If exploders do occur, attempt to remove all contaminated eggs. If problem is severe, empty machine, clean it and start again.

4 INFLUENCE OF NUTRITION ON HEALTH CONTROL

DAVID SPEIGHT BSc, Dipl. Ag.

Feeding of table poultry
Feeding of laying poultry
Nutrition and skeletal problems in poultry
Feed raw materials and poultry health
Moulds and mycotoxins
Quality control

The maintenance and promotion of good health is one of the major objectives in the nutrition of all farm livestock, including poultry. Without it the high levels of productivity and quality of the end product required to achieve good levels of profitability cannot be sustained and consequently health is a major consideration in determining the nutrient requirements of poultry.

The nutritional requirements of the chicken are probably the most highly researched of any species. It has provided the experimental animal for the discovery and investigation of the significance of many nutrients such as the vitamins and trace minerals. It has also been used to establish nutritional principles which have been extended into the nutrition of many other species, including humans.

The investigation of all stages of growth from the production of the egg, nutrition of the developing embryo and the requirements of the growing chicken for both egg and meat production for a wide range of nutrients means that the practical nutritionist has a very sound basis for the specification and formulation of feeds for all classes of poultry in all phases of production.

This considerable information base means that simple nutritional deficiencies are now very rare in practical poultry production situations. However, nutritional problems affecting the health of poultry still occur, but in general these are more complex and are usually related to specific situations.

A detailed description of the nutrient requirements of domestic poultry is outside the scope of this book and is well documented elsewhere in a number of authoritative published accounts based on this vast resource of research information. The intention here is only to give a broad outline of the nutritional requirements sufficient to illustrate the principles which lay behind the commercial feeding programmes for the major production phases of poultry production.

Feeding of table poultry

Feeding the broiler

The major part of the broiler industry in the UK is based on the production of a bird of 1.75–2.00 kg (3.75–4.4 lb) liveweight at 42–47 days of age although there is some more specialized production of poussins, weighing around 900 g (2 lb) and heavy chickens at up to 3 kg (6.6 lb) in liveweight.

Normally in the production of broilers the chickens are grown as hatched: i.e. the sexes are grown together with the normal distribution of males and females, although in some circumstances sexed growing is practised.

Feeding programme

The nutrient requirements of the broiler change significantly over the growing period, with the requirement for protein, amino acids and minerals reducing in relation to energy with increasing age. Normally protein and amino acid components of feeds are relatively expensive and therefore, from a nutritional point of view, a programme including three feeds with decreasing protein levels would be applied.

With the exception of a very small proportion of broilers grown under organic production programmes all broilers are fed feeds which contain cocci-diostats at prophylactic levels to control the intestinal parasitic disease, cocci-diosis. Additionally most feeds will also include a growth promoter. In Europe and the USA and in many other countries in the world controls on the use of feed additives require that these are withdrawn before slaughter, in order to ensure that the poultry products are free from residues. This means that a further ration is required in the growing programme, from which growth-promoting feed additives and prophylactic medication such as coccidiostats are withdrawn, to be fed for the five days prior to slaughter, making a total of four different feeds in the programme (Table 4.1). Feeds throughout the programme are fed ad lib to maximize growth.

Table 4.1 Feeding programme for the production of broilers

Feed	Feeding period (days)
Starter	0–11
Grower	11–28
Finisher	28–5 days prior to kill
Withdrawal	5 days prior to kill

The effects of feeding diets of higher energy levels to chickens is to increase broiler performance in terms of both liveweight and feed conversion rate (Jackson *et al.* 1982; Pesti and Smith 1984). The most important sources of supplementary energy available to the nutritionist to increase the nutrient density of the diet are lipids such as animal fats and vegetable oils.

The young chick, when changing from yolk sac nutrition to digestion of normal feed, has a limited ability to digest fat, particularly animal fats such as tallow (Krogdahl 1985). The choice of fats and their content in the starter feed is therefore limited, consequently the means of increasing the nutrient density of broiler starter formulations are very circumscribed.

As the bird gets older its lipid digestive system develops and there is more scope to formulate feeds to higher nutrient densities with higher supplementary fat levels. This is of some advantage in broiler feeding programmes, as research demonstrates that increasing energy levels through the feeding programme results in increased broiler performance (Newcombe and Summers 1984). With increasing age the broiler's requirement for protein and amino acids in relation to energy is reduced (Tables 4.2a, 4.2b).

Feed form

Feeds for broilers are normally pelleted in order to increase feed consumption and therefore rate of liveweight gain (Brue and Latshaw 1981; McNaughton and Reece 1982). Broiler starter feed is crumbled after pelleting to reduce the particle size for the young chick. The appropriate size for broiler pellets is 3 mm (⅛ in).

Sexed growing of broilers

Males grow faster than females, have a higher feed consumption and convert feed more efficiently at the same age. Females tend to be fatter than males. The result of these growth and performance differences is that the sexes have different nutrient requirements with the males having a higher requirement for protein and amino acids to support their higher growth rate, and the females needing a lower energy level to limit their fat deposition.

While the male is some 7% larger and has consumed some 7% more feed than the female by 14 days of age (Marks 1985), the nutrient requirements in the starter phase, from 0 to between 11 and 21 days, are not regarded as being sufficiently different to justify the production of separate starter feeds and both males and females receive the same formulation during this period.

The different requirements of the sexes in the grower and finisher periods can be met in one of two ways.

Table 4.2a Recommended ratios to ME (g/MJ/kg) for certain amino acids and major minerals in diets for growing broilers

	Feeding period		
	0–11 days	11–28 days	28 days to slaughter*
Crude protein	18.1	16.3	14.9
Lysine	0.96	0.85	0.70
Methionine	0.40	0.34	0.31
SAA	0.72	0.64	0.54
Tryptophan	0.18	0.17	0.13
Threonine	0.61	0.55	0.46
Calcium	0.85	0.75	0.65
Av. Phosphorus	0.35	0.33	0.30
Sodium	0.13	0.13	0.13
Chloride	0.12	0.12	0.12

Table 4.2b Recommended ratios to ME (Mcals/lb) for certain amino acids and major minerals in diets for growing broilers

	Feeding period		
	0–11 days	11–28 days	28 days to slaughter*
Crude protein	16.71	15.05	13.75
Lysine	0.89	0.78	0.65
Methionine	0.37	0.31	0.29
SAA	0.66	0.59	0.50
Tryptophan	0.17	0.16	0.12
Threonine	0.56	0.51	0.42
Calcium	0.78	0.69	0.60
Av. Phosphorus	0.32	0.30	0.28
Sodium	0.12	0.12	0.12
Chloride	0.11	0.11	0.11

* Broiler feeds will normally contain medicinal substances such as coccidiostats and growth promoters. It will normally be necessary to withdraw the medication from the feed for the periods appropriate to the substances incorporated prior to slaughter.

1. Feeds can be formulated separately to the nutrient specifications for each sex.
2. The same feeds can be used for both sexes but in different feeding programmes.

The second option involves a degree of compromise nutritionally as, while it fulfils the requirement of the female for feeds of a lower protein level at a lower age, under most circumstances it will involve the earlier introduction of feeds of a higher energy level. However, there are practical advantages in this method as it involves a smaller number of feeds to manufacture and manage on the farm.

While there is some potential advantage in exploiting the economies relating to the lower nutrient requirements of females when compared with those for males, unless the strain of broilers employed is one in which feather sexing is possible, this advantage is offset by the extra cost of sexing the day-old chick and the added stress imposed by this. The different housing requirements of the sexes in terms of stocking density may also create some complications in the optimum use of the production floor space available.

Situations where sexed growing is necessary are where the normal distribution of weight between the sexes does not meet the market requirement and, more specifically, when males are to be retained to be grown on to heavier weights in the production of heavy chickens or roasters (see below).

Feeding the roaster

While the production of roasters to oven-ready weights of 2–3 kg (4.4–6.6 lb) only accounts for a small proportion of the meat chicken market it is nonetheless significant as a specialist niche of production.

The production of heavy chickens or roasters usually involves growing the chickens on a sexed basis. The growth and feed conversion of males is superior to that of females and they have greater potential to grow to heavier weights. Also they tend not to deposit as much fat in the carcase. As is the case with sexed growing of chickens to the lower broiler weights, the sexes are often raised in sections of the same house until the females are taken out at normal broiler killing age. The males remaining to roaster weight are allowed the extra space to develop at a lower stocking density. In many cases both the males and the females will be served by the same feeding equipment in the house and therefore the same feeding regimen while they are housed together.

Roasters are normally marketed fresh and carcase quality in terms of finish and freedom from blemish is very important. One of the major problems leading to difficulties with carcase quality arises from leg weakness resulting in breast blisters and hock burn.

While the aetiology of leg weakness problems is complex and involves genotype, disease status and management of the chicken, some of these problems can be influenced by nutritional factors (Leeson and Summers 1988).

The early feeds in the feeding programmes for roasters are normally formulated to lower nutrient densities than those designed for broilers. Reduction in growth rate by restricting energy (Haye and Simons 1978) or restriction of protein in the early stages of growth (Hulan *et al.* 1980) has been demonstrated to reduce the incidence of leg weakness problems in broilers or roasters. The longer period of growth of the roaster allows the chicken to make up any deficiency in growth rate resulting from these lower specification starter feeds by compensatory growth.

The feeding programmes will usually consist of five feeds including a withdrawal feed (Table 4.3) from which all medication is omitted and which is fed for the 5 days prior to slaughter. The feeds contain reducing levels of protein and amino acids as the chickens get older.

Table 4.3 Feeding programme for the production of heavy roaster chickens

Feed	Feeding period (days)
Starter	0–14
Grower No. 1	14–28
Grower No. 2	28–49
Finisher	49–5 days prior to kill
Withdrawal	5 days prior to kill

All the feeds with the exception of the withdrawal feed will contain a coccidiostat and also, in most cases, a growth promoter.

Feeding the poussin

Poussins are another very specialized form of chicken production. Usually only males are utilized and a feeding programme using only three feeds—starter, grower and withdrawal feed—is applied. The formulation of these feeds is normally the same as those used for broiler production.

Feeding of laying poultry

Feeding the replacement pullet

The objectives of feeding systems for rearing chickens as pullet replacements for breeding or commercial egg production are different in some respects from those in rearing chickens for the table. While maximum growth rate consistent with the required carcase quality and cost of production is of supreme importance in the production of broilers, the most important objective in growing chickens as pullet replacements is that they should be physiologically well prepared to maximize the number of eggs produced in the case of the commercial egg layer, or the number and quality of chicks, in the case of the breeder hen.

Feeding the broiler breeder replacement pullet

Due to many years of intensive selection for high rates of liveweight gain and high levels of feed consumption, broiler strains of poultry have developed a marked propensity for over-consumption of feed leading to obesity when they are fed on an ad lib basis. This means that it has been necessary to develop feeding programmes which will restrict their energy intake and therefore the rate of weight gain of the bird. Feed restriction, together with a reduction in day length in controlled environment housing, also delays the development of sexual maturity of the bird.

A variety of methods have been tried to achieve this objective. Early attempts at feed restriction entailed dilution of the feed with inert materials or very low-energy ingredients such as oat-husk meal. These were generally unsuccessful due to the bird's ability to increase its feed intake to fulfil its energy requirement. Another feed formulation technique which was tried was to restrict the amount of protein in the feed (Waldroup et al. 1966; Harms et al. 1968), or to use a feed in which the amino acids were imbalanced (Singsen et al. 1964). These feeds were based on the principle that a deficiency of lysine depresses the feed intake of the bird and therefore reduces the rate of live-weight gain. This approach again only met with limited success largely due to lack of precision in the production of feeds with low protein and amino acid levels, as a result of the variability of raw materials, particularly cereals.

Ultimately it has been necessary to accept that the only method which permits sufficient control over the growth of the replacement broiler breeder pullet is to physically restrict the amount of feed the bird receives to that which will produce the required growth pattern; this is now the technique universally used in feeding broiler breeder pullet replacements. There are two ways in which this restricted amount of feed is allocated to the rearing flock:

1. Skip-a-day feeding in which the amount of feed required for two days is fed on alternate days and only a small grain scratch feed is fed on the none-feed day.
2. Daily feeding in which, as the name suggests, the birds receive their restricted allocation of feed on a daily basis.

The reasoning behind the skip-a-day technique (Voitle et al. 1974) is that the increased allocation of feed created by feeding two days' feed in one results in more uniform feed intake in the flock, enabling socially less-dominant birds greater opportunity to consume their share in relation to their more aggressive neighbours. There is, however, now some concern from the point of view of animal welfare at the deprivation of food on the 'off' feed days and current recommendations are moving towards daily feeding with the feed given in a single allocation per day, preferably in the early morning.

All the primary breeders of broiler stock produce recommendations for target weights for ages through the rearing period to 18–20 weeks of age for their own strains of chickens, and programmes of feed allocation to achieve these weights. The feeding programmes are presented as a guide and flock managers are advised to adjust these in relation to regular check weighings of pullets in order to ensure that the flock is maintained on the recommended growth curve.

Feed for rearing broiler breeders has traditionally been supplied as meal but in view of increasing concern regarding protection of flocks from salmonella infection there is a developing trend to textured feed in the form of unscreened crumbs manufactured from pellets prepared from heat-conditioned meal.

From a nutritional point of view the feeding programme for broiler breeder females utilizes a two- or three-feed programme consisting of a starter feed applied from 0 to 6 weeks, followed by a grower feed from 6 weeks to housing at point of lay (Table 4.4). As maximum liveweight gain is not a priority, feeds for rearing pullet replacements are usually lower in nutrient density than those for broilers. Typical levels of specification for the principal nutrients are shown in Table 4.5.

Table 4.4 Feeding programme for pullet rearing

Feed	Medication	Feeding period (weeks)
Starter	C*	0–6
Grower	C*	6–16
Grower No. 2		16–point of lay

C = Coccidiostat. The coccidiostat is normally included at a reducing level through the feeding programme to stimulate the development of immunity to coccidiosis.

Coccidiosis control

In contrast to the almost total control of coccidiosis required in broiler production the objective in coccidiosis control in the rearing of breeders is to allow some exposure to the coccidia. With most coccidiostats this means incorporating the coccidiostat at levels lower than those necessary for full coccidiosis control. Most coccidiostat programmes for pullet rearing recommend the incorporation of the drug at the full control level in the starter feed with a

Table 4.5 Recommended levels of crude protein, lysine, sulphur amino acids and major minerals in diets for rearing replacement pullets

	Feeding period	
	0–6 weeks Starter	6 weeks to pol Grower
ME(MJ/kg)	11.50	11.00
Crude Protein %	18.50	15.00
Lysine %	0.86	0.60
Methionine %	0.33	0.28
SAA %	0.65	0.50
Calcium %	1.00	1.00
Av. Phosphorus %	0.35	0.33
Salt (NaCl) %	0.37	0.37

reduced level in the first phase of feeding of the grower feed. This exposure at lower levels of the coccidiostat allows the pullet's immunity to coccidiosis to develop before she comes into egg production, when infection with the disease is much more damaging.

The requirement to incorporate a prophylactic coccidiostat in the system in the early stages of rearing means that the feeding system becomes a three-feed system, as the coccidiostat is required during the earlier part of the grower period and is withdrawn towards the end of rearing.

Methods of coccidiosis control other than the prophylactic inclusion of coccidiostats have been used with some success.

Live coccidial vaccines are used in broiler breeder rearing flocks in some parts of the world, particularly in the USA and Canada. At the present time considerable research effort is being applied to the development of genetically engineered monoclonal antibodies against coccidiosis, but none of these is yet on the market.

Some operators have attempted rearing replacements without any prophylactic treatment, waiting until the flock shows signs of infection and then treating the coccidiosis outbreak therapeutically at an early stage. While this method of control can be successful and results in a good level of immunity in the flock it requires extremely diligent management if serious damaging outbreaks are to be avoided.

Feeding the replacement broiler breeder male

Broiler breeder cockerels are best reared separately from the pullets in order to achieve better control of feed intake and liveweight. If the cockerels become too heavy, mating and fertility problems occur.

Research has shown that males can be reared successfully without any prejudice to their subsequent breeding performance on diets as low in protein as 12% (Vaughters *et al.* 1987; Wilson *et al.* 1987). However, from the point of view of commercial expediency they are normally fed on the same feed regime as the pullets. Breeders of broiler strain birds normally provide specific feeding and liveweight guides for their males.

Feeding the broiler breeder during lay

The broiler breeder pullets are normally transferred to their laying accommodation at about 18 weeks of age when the males are introduced to the flock and the feed is changed from the grower feed to a breeder layer diet. The laying feed is balanced for egg production, contains an increased calcium level and is supplemented to meet the needs of the developing embryo in the hatching egg (Table 4.6). The feed restriction policy which was essential during rearing

Table 4.6 Recommended levels of crude protein, lysine, sulphur amino acids and major minerals in diets for commercial layers and broiler breeders

	Layer	Broiler breeder
ME (MJ/kg)	11.50	11.50
Crude Protein %	16.00	15.50
Lysine %	0.62	0.55
Methionine %	0.28	0.30
SAA %	0.52	0.59
Calcium %	3.50	2.80
Av. Phosphorus %	0.35	0.33
Salt (NaCl) %	0.37	0.40

needs to be continued during lay but the allocation of feed is increased. The rate of increase of daily feed allowance is accelerated from about 15 weeks old in order to allow development of the bird towards sexual maturity. The short day length under which the birds have been reared is gradually increased week by week from 19 weeks old, to reach 14 hours at 24 weeks of age. This, along with the increase in feed allocation, brings the flock to sexual maturity and egg production in a controlled way.

As flock egg production increases the feed allowance is increased to reach about 455 kcal (1.905 MJ)/bird/day at peak egg production at about 32 weeks old. Peak production of egg mass/day occurs slightly later than egg number/day, at about 34 weeks. As egg mass production declines the feed allocation is gradually reduced at a rate of 2–3 kcal/bird/day each week (see page 185).

Feeding the commercial layer replacement pullet

In contrast with the broiler strain breeders the commercial layer breeds have been selected for a high level of egg production rather than maximum rate of body weight gain. This means that they do not have the same tendencies to over-consumption of energy and consequent obesity that is characteristic of broiler breeders and they can be fed ad lib throughout the rearing period. The feeds employed during rearing are similar to those described above for the broiler breeder.

Coccidiosis control is similar, with a step-down system of incorporation of a coccidiostat with the objective of establishing immunity against the disease. This is necessary as, even when the commercial layer is intensively housed in cages during the laying period, infection with coccidia can occur.

As in the case of the broiler breeder pullet the birds are reared under a restricted day length of about 8 hours to point of lay at 18 weeks old.

Feeding the commercial layer

Throughout lay the commercial egg layer is normally fed ad lib. The feeds used are usually of higher nutrient density than those used for feeding broiler breeder hens. The feeds are supplemented with calcium to fulfil the requirements of shell formation at the high rate of egg production of the modern commercial layer and to maintain its skeletal integrity. In the physiological process of egg shell formation the laying hen mobilizes calcium from its skeleton on a daily basis. If the calcium supply is deficient egg production is reduced or will cease. In some circumstances if the supply of calcium in the diet is very deficient the bird will suffer from a form of osteoporosis described as cage layer fatigue—the bird becomes paralysed and may die.

Egg yolk colour is an important factor in egg production and this is dependent on the supply of carotenoid pigments in the diet (Figure 4.1). These can be obtained from some raw materials such as maize (corn) or maize by-products such as maize gluten meal or dried green crops, e.g. dried grass or lucerne (alfalfa) meal. However, these sources of pigmentation are not always available or they may be economically unattractive; they are also rather variable and it is often necessary to supplement the feed with synthetic carotenoids in order to ensure that the eggs produced are of the required yolk colour.

Egg shell quality

Good egg shell quality is extremely important in the economics of egg

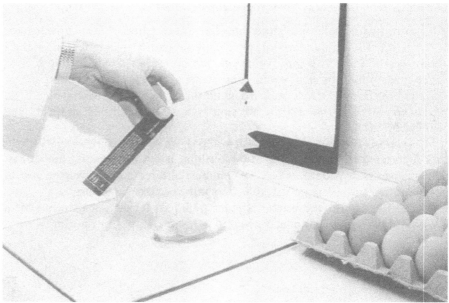

Figure 4.1 Measuring the yolk colour of eggs using the Roche colour fan.

production and losses between production and the consumer as a result of cracked and broken eggs have been estimated at between 6% and 8% (Washburn 1982). The factors involved in egg shell damage have been reviewed by Hamilton *et al.* (1980) and Washburn (1982). The extent of egg shell damage is dependent on the strength of the shell and its subsequent treatment.

Egg shell strength is influenced by mineral and vitamin nutrition and the age of the hen. Nutritional factors which have been implicated include vitamin D, calcium and phosphorus metabolism and electrolyte balance (Figure 4.2).

Calcium is the most important mineral element in egg shell formation. The egg shell contains 2.1 g of calcium leading to a requirement of 3.5 g/day (Miles 1981). With a daily feed consumption of around 100 g/day the calcium requirement in the feed is therefore 3.5%. The metabolism of calcium is controlled by endocrine systems involving oestrogens, calcitonin and a derivative of vitamin D_3 (1,25-dihydroxycholecalciferol).

Severe deficiencies of calcium will result in the hen ceasing egg production, while in the case of more moderate deficiency egg production is reduced. Deficiency in calcium content of the diet reduces shell weight and the proportion of calcium in the shell (Gilbert *et al.* 1981).

The content of phosphorus in the egg shell is very low in relation to that of calcium, at about 20 mg (Miles 1981). Some researchers have claimed that reductions in dietary phosphorus levels from normal levels of 600–700 mg/day have resulted in improvements in egg shell quality although other workers

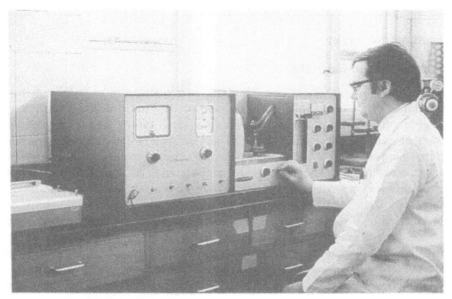

Figure 4.2 Analysis of minerals in feeds using an atomic absorption spectrophotometer.

have failed to demonstrate this effect. Excessive levels of phosphorus have, however, been shown to reduce egg shell quality (El-Boushy 1979; Miles and Harms 1982; Miles *et al.* 1983; Roland and Farmer 1986). The recommended level of inclusion in feed is 0.35% of non-phytin phosphorus.

In recent years, following work by Mongin (1968), attention has been focused on the effects of electrolyte balance on egg shell quality on the basis that in the process of shell formation the deposition of calcium carbonate is dependent upon blood pH and is depressed in conditions of metabolic acidosis at low levels of blood pH. Research has shown that metabolic acidosis can be produced by increasing the ratio of chloride to sodium in the diet (Cohen *et al.* 1972). There are several reports in the literature demonstrating that egg shell thickness and shell strength was improved if part of the dietary requirement for sodium is satisfied by supplementing the diet with sodium bicarbonate. This leads to a reduction in the chloride level as a consequence of lowered inclusion of salt (sodium chloride), although some workers in the field could not confirm this effect. Mongin (1980a) showed that supplementation of the diet with sodium bicarbonate to increase the value of Na + K − Cl to 200 meg/kg or more, resulted in significant improvements in shell quality.

Feeding the turkey

Feeding the growing turkey

The market for turkeys in the UK requires a wide range in weight. It has developed from the highly seasonal trade of the turkey for the Christmas celebration, to a market which supplies the small turkey sold on a week by week basis to the housewife forming part of her weekly decision making in her purchasing of the weekend roast and the large turkey required by the catering trade. In addition to the whole bird trade, a market is developing for turkey joints and for convenience prepared turkey recipe products. These are usually produced from large turkeys in order to take account of the economy of production of these larger birds. In the turkey there is a marked degree of sexual dimorphism with the males being about twice the size of the females at maturity. In commercial production this means that the female hen turkeys are slaughtered to fulfil the market requirements for the lower weights, while the demand for heavy turkeys is met by growing on male stag turkeys from genetically large strains.

In contrast to the broiler which is normally slaughtered at 6–7 weeks old at about 2.2 kg, the heavy turkey may be grown for 20–24 weeks to reach a market weight of about 20 kg. As a result of the significant changes in nutrient requirements over the long feeding period, feeding programmes for growing turkeys consist of a relatively large number of feeds with many programmes changing feed on a monthly basis throughout the growing period. In other programmes the feed changes are made at more frequent intervals in the early stages of growth, when the requirements are changing more rapidly than towards the end of the growing period when the changes are less dramatic. The starting poult's requirement for protein, or more correctly amino acids, is much higher than for the starting chicken at approximately 30% compared with about 23% in the case of the chicken. This difference is related to the very high rate of protein deposition and low rate of fat deposition in the turkey in comparison with the chicken. In a similar manner to that described for the chicken, the requirement for protein and amino acids in relation to energy declines with age (Tables 4.7a, 4.7b).

In order to satisfy the wide range of carcase weights required by the market, feeding programmes must be designed which will ensure that a desirable carcase quality is achieved by the time the turkey reaches slaughter age. An important physiological difference between the growing turkey and the chicken is that it does not show the same propensity to deposit depot fats. At normal slaughter weights therefore there is no problem of excess carcase fat. Indeed at the lower weights and ages it is particularly important to ensure that the diet is high enough in energy to allow sufficient fat deposition to ensure a

Table 4.7a Recommended ratios to ME (MJ/kg) for certain amino acids and major minerals in diets for growing turkeys*

	Feeding period						
	0–2	2–5	5–8	8–11	11–14	14–18	18–24
Lysine	1.55	1.39	1.21	1.01	0.87	0.70	0.59
Methionine	0.54	0.49	0.43	0.37	0.33	0.29	0.27
SAA	0.94	0.87	0.79	0.71	0.65	0.60	0.58
Tryptophan	0.26	0.23	0.20	0.17	0.14	0.11	0.09
Threonine	0.98	0.90	0.82	0.70	0.56	0.45	0.40
Calcium	1.15	1.10	1.00	0.95	0.90	0.80	0.70
Av. Phosphorus	0.70	0.65	0.60	0.55	0.50	0.45	0.40
Salt (NaCl)	0.32	0.29	0.20	0.29	0.28	0.28	0.28

Table 4.7b Recommended ratios to ME (Mcal/lb) for certain amino acids and major minerals in diets for growing turkeys*

	Feeding period						
	0–2	2–5	5–8	8–11	11–14	14–18	18–24
Lysine	1.43	1.28	1.12	0.93	0.80	0.65	0.54
Methionine	0.50	0.45	0.40	0.34	0.30	0.27	0.25
SAA	0.87	0.80	0.73	0.66	0.60	0.55	0.54
Tryptophan	0.24	0.21	0.18	0.16	0.13	0.10	0.08
Threonine	0.90	0.83	0.76	0.65	0.52	0.42	0.37
Calcium	1.06	1.02	0.92	0.88	0.83	0.74	0.65
Av. Phosphorus	0.65	0.60	0.55	0.51	0.46	0.42	0.37
Salt (NaCl)	0.30	0.27	0.27	0.27	0.26	0.26	0.26

* Turkey feeds will normally contain medicinal substances such as coccidiostats, anti-blackhead drugs and growth promoters. It will normally be necessary to withdraw the medication from the feed for the periods appropriate to the substances incorporated prior to slaughter.

satisfactory level of carcase finish. This is usually achieved by the addition of supplementary dietary fat.

Feed form

Feed form is very important in feeding turkeys and they respond well to feed in the form of good quality pellets with a low content of fines in terms of feed intake and liveweight gain. Nixey (1989) found that starting poults fed crumbs were 16% heavier at 7 days old and 2.3.% heavier at 28 days of age than poults fed mash. In normal commercial practice therefore turkeys are fed crumbs in the starter period followed by pellets through the rest of the programme.

Medication

Turkeys are susceptible to two important parasitic infections which are controlled prophylactically by feed medication. Like chickens, the young turkey poult can become infected with coccidiosis although the coccidial species are different. The most important turkey species are *Eimeria adenoeides* and *E. meleagrimitis*. To control coccidiosis feeds for turkeys up to about 8 weeks old are normally medicated with an approved coccidiostat. The other important parasitic infection of turkeys is blackhead. This disease affects turkeys at a later stage of growth and is controlled by prophylactic incorporation of an anti-blackhead drug. These drugs must be withdrawn from the feed for the prescribed period before the turkeys are slaughtered for human consumption, hence it is necessary to utilize a withdrawal feed in the feeding programme for market turkeys. The recommended medication programme for turkeys through the growing period is shown in Table 4.8.

Table 4.8 Recommended medication for feeds for growing turkeys

	Feeding period						
	0–2	2–5	5–8	8–11	11–14	14–18	18–24
Coccidiostat	+	+	+	+	−	−	−
Anti-blackhead	+	+	+	+	+	+	+
Growth promoter	+	+	+	+	+	+	+

Note: It is necessary to feed a withdrawal feed prior to slaughter for the period prescribed for the drugs included if the finisher feed being fed at the end of the feeding programme contains a coccidiostat, anti-blackhead drug, or growth promoter.

Feeding the turkey breeder

Feeding during the rearing period

In contrast to the broiler breeder female which becomes obese if she is fed ad lib and therefore has to be subjected to a relatively high level of feed restriction if her subsequent reproductive performance is not to be jeopardized, the turkey breeder female does not respond well to feed restriction during rearing. Many studies have shown that there is no advantage to be gained from restriction during the rearing period and in some cases resulted in reductions in egg output have been recorded (Touchburn *et al.* 1968; Jones *et al.* 1976; Kreuger *et al.* 1978). In normal commercial practice turkey replacement breeders are fed ad lib throughout the rearing period.

Feeds for rearing replacement breeders can be formulated to the most cost effective level of energy as no advantage has been demonstrated in feeding diets at a high energy level (Potter and Leighton 1973).

Feeding programmes used in commercial practice usually follow a similar pattern to those for market turkeys up to approximately 12 weeks of age, when a relatively low protein developer diet is introduced and is fed until they are housed in the production accommodation and the daylength is increased. This usually means that the turkeys are reared on a four-stage programme. Feeds fed to approximately 8 weeks old will normally contain a coccidiostat and an anti-blackhead drug will be included up to point of lay.

Feeding during lay

While the broiler hen during lay has to continue to be maintained on a restricted feeding regime, the turkey breeder behaves physiologically in a completely different way. At the onset of egg production her feed intake falls and her body weight reduces dramatically even though she is offered an ad lib feeding regime. Later her feed intake recovers and increases to the end of lay. Whitehead (1989) showed that the loss in bodyweight is due almost completely to a reduction in body fat level. The changes in bodyweight do not seem to be responsive to nutritional manipulation and the loss in bodyweight does not appear to be associated with any reduction in production.

The egg mass produced by the breeder turkey is relatively much lower than that of the laying hen. As a result the turkey breeder diet can be formulated at a lower level of protein and lower calcium level than is the case with the hen (Table 4.9).

Table 4.9 Recommended levels of crude protein, lysine, sulphur amino acids and major minerals in diets for turkey breeders

	Turkey breeder
ME (MJ/kg)	12.00
Crude Protein %	15.00
Lysine %	0.65
Methionine %	0.30
SAA %	0.55
Calcium %	2.50
Av. Phosphorus %	0.40
Salt (NaCl) %	0.40

Nutrition and skeletal problems in poultry

The most important skeletal problems in poultry relate to leg abnormalities, with a number of conditions occurring particularly in intensively managed poultry.

Leg problems are a cause of considerable economic loss to the poultry industry, particularly in the poultry meat sector where both broilers and turkeys are affected. Leg abnormalities result in lameness, which inevitably leads the affected bird to spend a greater part of its time resting on the litter. In many cases this causes damage to the skin of the bird due to pressure-induced necrosis or contact dermatitis in the form of breast blisters, hock burn or scabby hip syndrome. This is also often associated with depression in liveweight.

The aetiology of these leg abnormalities is complex and is not confined to aspects of nutrition. Genetics, disease, environmental factors and management are also implicated. However, a variety of nutrients have been implicated in leg abnormalities.

Energy and protein

Haye and Simons (1978) concluded that energy restriction in early growth will substantially reduce leg problems in broilers. Hulan *et al.* (1980) found that reduction in protein level of the diet early in development reduced leg abnormalities in roaster chickens. Edwards and Sorenson (1987) restricted young broilers' access to feed for 8–10 hours per day and demonstrated a reduced incidence of the leg disorder tibial dyschondroplasia. These reports suggest that restriction in body weight, by reducing the plane of nutrition, will alleviate the incidence of leg weakness and they therefore imply that the cause of the problem is the achievement of excessive body weight on a skeleton which cannot support it. Leeson and Summers (1988) suggest, however, that the situation is more complex than this and that nutrient interrelationships may be more important, such as interference of high protein levels with the metabolism of the B vitamin folic acid or imbalances between amino acids and non-protein nitrogen in the diet.

Vitamins

Deficiencies in a number of vitamins have been associated with leg disorders. The classical condition of nutritional rickets involves deficiency of vitamin D. Perosis is associated with choline or nicotinic acid (niacin) deficiency along with other factors including the trace element manganese. Deficiency of biotin in the breeder diet has also been shown to cause skeletal deformity including perosis in newly hatched chicks (Couch *et al.* 1948). Nicotinic acid deficiency also causes bowing of the legs and enlargement of the tibiotarsal joint. The involvement of vitamin B_6 (pyridoxine) in tibial dyschondroplasia has been demonstrated (Bierne and Jensen 1981).

Vitamin D

Nutritional rickets is one of the classical skeletal problems associated with nutritional deficiency. It occurs in young chicks and the signs are weakness of the legs and claws and a rubbery beak. On post-mortem the ribs show a characteristic beading. Growth is also impaired. The cause of nutritional rickets is a deficiency of vitamin D or deficiencies of calcium or phosphorus in the diet.

Very high dietary levels of vitamin A have also resulted in an incidence of rickets suggesting that excesses of this vitamin may interfere with the absorption or metabolism of vitamin D. It should be noted, however, that the levels of vitamin A causing this problem are far higher than the normal practical levels of supplementation with this vitamin for poultry.

Not all cases of rickets are the result of feed deficiencies of vitamin D. More recently a condition known as field rickets has been recognized in turkeys (Hurwitz *et al.* 1973; Walser *et al.* 1980; Olson *et al.* 1981; Bar *et al.* 1987). This disorder resembles classical nutritional rickets in many respects but it occurs in diets which are more than adequate in vitamin D_3 and does not respond to injections of this vitamin. It is thought that the condition results from genetic defects in the metabolism of vitamin D.

Nicotinic acid (niacin)

Deficiency of nicotinic acid results in bowing of the legs and enlargement of the hocks in young poultry, which may lead to perosis. Turkey poults, ducklings and pheasant chicks have a higher requirement than chickens for nicotinic acid and are therefore more likely to show signs of deficiency. There is a nutritional interrelationship between nicotinic acid and the amino acid tryptophan, and nicotinic acid deficiency signs are more likely on diets which are marginal in tryptophan. The synthesis of nicotinic acid from tryptophan also depends on adequate levels of vitamin B_6 (pyridoxine) being present in the diet.

Naturally occurring nicotinic acid in the ingredients of the diet is often present in a bound form which is unavailable to the bird. It is normal practice therefore to supplement the feed to the full requirement level.

Vitamin B₆ (pyridoxine)

Apart from its possible involvement in nicotinic acid deficiency as described above, vitamin B_6 has been implicated in leg abnormalities by Greis and Scott (1972). Bierne and Jensen (1981) experienced a high incidence of twisted legs in their research programmes although the diet was supplemented with vitamin B_6, and they carried out a study to investigate whether increased levels of vitamin B_6 would reduce the level of this condition. Although the very high levels of supplementation applied by these workers reduced the incidence to some degree they concluded that vitamin B_6 is not the only cause of twisted legs and that other factors are also involved in this abnormality.

Biotin

Biotin deficiency in turkeys or chicks causes a characteristic dermatitis of the soles of the feet. This develops into cracks of the skin which then haemorrhage and often become infected and ulcerated, particularly if the litter on which the birds are housed is wet (Harms and Simpson 1977). This infection of the feet causes the bird to rest on its hocks with the result that the birds often suffer from hock burn and breast blisters (Harms and Simpson 1975; Martland 1985). In addition to these signs biotin deficiency will cause enlargement of the hocks.

Minerals

Minerals play a key role in the development of the skeleton and maintenance of its integrity. Calcium and phosphorus are the major elements in the mineral structure of the skeleton and their role in relation to leg disorders, particularly in tibial dyschondroplasia, has been studied by a number of researchers. Calcium and phosphorus balance is important in the aetiology of leg weakness. Edwards and Veltmann (1983) showed that high phosphorus and low calcium levels were associated with a high incidence of tibial dyschondroplasia. They also failed to demonstrate that the incidence of this condition was related to the level of retention of either calcium or phosphorus or to the percentage of bone ash, a factor which has often been used as an index of calcium and phosphorus adequacy in the investigation of the requirements of these elements. Hulan et al. (1986) found that increasing the ratio of calcium to available phosphorus from 1.75 to 2.65 in the starter feed (fed from 0–21 days), and from 3.02 to

3.55 in the finisher phase (22–40 days) reduced the incidence of both tibial dyschondroplasia and other leg abnormalities, but also reduced the biological performance of the chickens. The relationship of high phosphorus level with a high incidence of tibial dyschondroplasia was confirmed by Edwards (1988), who also found that high calcium levels were associated with a reduced incidence of the disorder.

This research demonstrates the importance of the balance of calcium and phosphorus in the diet of the chicken. In particular it suggests that high levels of available phosphorus may lead to increased incidences of leg abnormalities in the broiler chicken.

Acid–base balance

It has been postulated that acid–base balance is an important factor in the aetiology of leg abnormalities in poultry, based on the findings of Leach and Neisheim (1965) that cation:anion relationships influenced the incidence of tibial dyschondroplasia. Sauveur and Mongin (1978) found that excess of chloride caused metabolic acidosis which was associated with an increase in the incidence of tibial dyschondroplasia and that this could be corrected by supplementation with sodium or potassium. Mongin (1980b) addressed the problem of cation:anion ratio and balance and expressed $(Na + K) - Cl$ as milliequivalents per $100\,g$ of diet. He concluded that this factor should be $250\,meq/100\,g$ for the chicken.

Since this work was published there have been a number of other investigations into the role of electrolytes in poultry performance and their influence on the incidence of leg abnormalities. Nelson et al. (1981) studied the effect of altering the dietary cation and anion content of the diet on chick performance and concluded that the incidence of crooked legs was reduced when the cation:anion ratio was widened by the addition of magnesium to change the cation level and of phosphorus to alter the anion level. Hulan et al. (1987) investigated the effects of cation:anion balance and calcium on broiler performance and leg abnormalities and concluded that increasing the levels of dietary sodium, potassium or calcium in relation to chloride decreased the incidence of tibial dyschondroplasia, but that they were interdependent on each other. Halley et al. (1987) investigated the possible involvement of calcium, magnesium, phosphorus and sulphate and concluded that widening the cation:anion ratio with calcium or magnesium reduced the incidence of tibial dyschondroplasia while narrowing it with chloride, phosphorus or sulphate increased it.

Clearly the involvement of minerals in the aetiology of leg abnormalities is complex and the correct balance of these is very important in the control of leg disorders, particularly in table poultry.

Feed raw materials and poultry health

The choice of raw materials for the formulation and manufacture of feeds is generally dictated by local availability and economics. The cost of feed is the major item in the production of poultry products and accounts for 70–80% of the total cost of production, hence it is very important that the cost of feed should be minimized to an extent consistent with the optimal performance of the stock.

Many of the feed ingredients for poultry are simple plant or animal products which are produced specifically as feed ingredients or have been subjected to a minimum of processing, being the by-products of human food manufacture.

While feed raw materials are often considered primarily as sources of a particular nutrient most of them contribute a wide range of nutrients including energy in the form of carbohydrates or fats, proteins and their constituent amino acids, minerals and vitamins, the major difference being in the relative proportions of nutrients in each source. For example cereals contain low proportions of protein and amino acids and high proportions of energy in the form of carbohydrates, i.e. starch, while in the case of oilseed by-products or animal by-products the opposite is the case.

Values are well documented for the nutrient components of most of the available feed ingredients based on standard methodology, and these provide a sound basis for the formulation of feeds against comprehensively researched nutritional requirement data for the various classes of poultry at their different stages of production.

Feed ingredients may be conveniently classified into the following broad categories:

- Cereals and cereal by-products
- Other energy ingredients
- Vegetable proteins
- Animal proteins
- Minerals
- Vitamins

Cereals

The choice of cereals, which are the major source of nutrients in the diet in most circumstances, is often determined by which cereals are produced locally. Thus poultry feeds in the USA are usually based on maize (corn) while in northern Europe wheat is generally used as the cereal choice. This factor has led to different market preferences for aspects of poultry quality in different parts of the world, particularly with regard to skin colour of chickens, with a preference for yellow chickens in regions where maize has been the cereal most readily available, and white-fleshed chickens where traditionally feeds have been based on wheat. Other cereals such as sorghum (milo), barley, oats, rice, rye or triticale can be fed to poultry where they are locally available at competitive prices.

There are few problems associated with cereal grains which are detrimental to growth, production or general health of poultry.

Maize (corn)

Maize is very widely used throughout the world as a poultry feed, except in poultry meat production where the market requires white-skinned birds; it is relatively free from problems associated with anti-nutritional factors. It can therefore be fed without limit in feeds for poultry in all circumstances except where markets demand poultry products free from pigmentation. Maize and its by-products are good sources of carotenoid pigments where these are required in feeds for either egg yolk coloration or in the production of yellow-skinned chickens. It has the highest energy value of any of the cereals used in poultry production and a significant level of oil which has a high content of the essential fatty acid, linoleic acid.

Wheat

Wheat is widely used as a base cereal in diets for all classes of poultry and is preferred over barley or oats because of its higher energy content, which usually makes it more economically attractive than these other cereals. As in the case of maize it is also reasonably free from nutritional problems and can be fed without limit in poultry feeds. It is relatively high in protein and therefore makes an important contribution to amino acid nutrition when it is used as the base cereal.

Wheat is, however, relatively deficient in biotin (vitamin H) and the bio-availability of that which is present is poor. Feeds in which this is the major cereal may result in signs of biotin deficiency if they are not adequately supplemented. In young chicks a marginal deficiency of biotin may lead to fatty liver and kidney syndrome (FLKS). The involvement of biotin in this syndrome was demonstrated by Whitehead and Blair (1974) and Whitehead et al. (1975). The aetiology of the disease is complex and research has shown that factors other than the biotin level in the diet affect the occurrence of FLKS.

Biotin deficiency in older chicks or turkeys results in loose feathering and dermatitis, with cracking of the skin on the soles of the feet; these cracks remain open and haemorrhagic and may become infected. Swollen hocks and bowed legs are also caused by biotin deficiency.

Modern diets are normally adequately supplemented with biotin and deficiencies are rarely seen.

Sorghum

Sorghum grain is grown widely in many areas of the world. There are a number of grain types including milo, kaffir corn, dari and durra. Grain types vary in colour from yellow through brown to purple and the dark-coloured grains contain tannins at levels which may reduce their palatability (Mangan 1988). Some varieties have been bred for bird resistance. However, the yellow varieties of milo are well accepted by poultry and sorghum is the second most important feed grain in the USA. The grain does not contain any effective levels of pigmenting xanthophylls and therefore can be used as a substitute for wheat in the production of white-skinned broilers.

Barley

Barley is a very important feed grain in more temperate climates. It is of lower energy value than the other feed grains as it retains its hull after harvest. As a result the price of barley needs to be at a significant discount to wheat to be economically attractive in poultry feed formulations.

Barley contains significant levels of a complex carbohydrate, β-glucan, which is not readily digestible by the chicken and causes wet droppings. This limits the amount of barley which can be included in formulations as, when birds are reared on litter, wet droppings can result in problems such as pododermatitis or coccidiosis, or in the case of caged layers to problems of litter handling in automated systems. A significant amount of research effort has been applied to the development of suitable β-glucanase enzyme preparations which will survive feed processing, and some of these are now coming onto the market (Hesselman et al. 1981).

Rye

In some European countries rye is grown in significant quantities and a considerable proportion of this is used for animal feeding. It typically contains a lower level of protein than wheat but has a more favourable amino acid profile. The nutrient digestibility of rye is lower than that of wheat and this therefore results in this cereal having a lower metabolizable energy level. Its use in poultry feeding is limited by the anti-nutritive factors with which it is associated (Jeroch 1987). The major factor suggested for the poor nutritive value of rye is its content of indigestible non-starch carbohydrates, including soluble and insoluble pentosans and pectins, which poultry cannot digest as they do not produce the necessary enzymes. These carbohydrates depress the digestibility of other nutrients and, in addition, because of their water-binding capacity and viscosity they produce sticky wet faeces which cause management and carcase quality problems in meat poultry and dirty down-graded eggs in laying hens. As with barley there is current research interest in the development of feed enzyme systems which will overcome these problems. Other anti-nutritive factors identified in rye are tannins, alkyl-resorcinols and trypsin inhibitors which interfere with the digestion of protein. The use of rye is therefore very limited in poultry diets.

Triticale

Triticale is a hybrid cereal produced by crossing wheat with rye. It has been developed with the objectives of producing a high-yielding cereal which would perform well on poorer soil types and which would combine the higher protein levels of wheat with the favourable amino acid composition of rye. The protein and amino acid levels of triticale vary considerably between varieties (Charmley and Greenhalgh 1987). The lysine content as a proportion of the total protein has been found to be intermediate between that of wheat and rye. The energy content is also very variable between varieties. Some varieties of triticale also show the characteristics of rye in their content of anti-nutritional factors and this limits their use in poultry diets (Rudgren 1988; Jeroch 1987).

Cereal by-products

Most cereals grown for the human food market undergo some processing in their preparation for their eventual food role. In most cases this entails the removal of the various seed coat components by dry milling processes—to produce husk meals in the case of oats, rice and barley, and bran fractions in the case of wheat and rice. These products are low in energy in comparison to the original cereals from which they are derived. Their use is mainly confined to inclusion in diets for growing layer replacements, layers or breeders. The bran fractions are usually higher in protein than the original cereals and they can make a useful contribution to fulfilling the amino acid requirements in appropriate diets.

In the case of maize, while some dry milling products are available, others are produced by wet milling in the production of starch. This process produces a low-energy bran fraction—maize gluten feed—and a higher energy product resulting from the wet separation of the gluten from the starch and subsequent drying—maize gluten meal. This latter is a high-protein, high-energy material which is also very high in the xanthophyll maize pigments. It is therefore a valuable source of supplementary pigmentation in diets for layers or yellow-skinned broilers.

Generally the cereal milling by-products are free from nutritional problems. An exception to this is full-fat rice bran, which may be subject to oxidative rancidity as a result of the highly unsaturated oil which it contains. This may result in deleterious effects on any vitamins subject to oxidation, such as vitamin E.

Other energy ingredients

Other energy ingredients available include the tropical tuber products such as cassava (tapioca or manioc) and sweet potato (Szylit *et al.* 1978). The by-products of the sugar industry, cane and beet molasses, are also sources of energy which are commercially available for use in feedstuffs.

Cassava

Cassava (*Manihot esculenta*) is widely grown in tropical areas and produces a high yield of starch which is used for both human and animal food. It needs to be processed very carefully to remove the glucoside linamarin, which is contained in the raw root. This glucoside liberates hydrocyanic acid on hydrolysis causing inhibition of thyroid activity. Cassava is very low in protein, at about 2.0%, but it can be high in ash due to residual contaminating sand. The product may also contain residual levels of hydrocyanic acid and oxalic acid. These can cause mild scouring. Cassava is very low in vitamins and trace minerals and this should be recognized when supplementing feeds containing this product. It can be included in broiler or layer feeds up to levels of 15–20%.

Sweet potato

Sweet potato (*Ipomoea batatas*) is another widely grown tropical tuber crop which until recently was primarily produced for human consumption; in some parts of the world surpluses are now available for processing as livestock feed. The product is very similar in composition to cassava and is a high-energy low-protein material. It has a similar metabolizable energy level to cassava but is free from the anti-nutritional factors found in cassava and can be included in poultry feeds at similar levels.

Molasses

Molasses is a by-product of the manufacture of sucrose from either sugar cane or sugar beet and contains approximately 50% sugars. It contains a very low level of protein at 2–4% and a relatively high level of ash. The potassium content is high and this leads to problems with wet droppings if excessive levels are used. The level of inclusion of molasses in poultry feeds is therefore limited to 3–4%.

Vegetable proteins

The most commonly used plant proteins in poultry feeds are soyabean meal, sunflower meal, cottonseed meal, rapeseed meal and maize gluten meal, although other vegetable proteins such as groundnut meal, safflower seed meal and sesame seed meal are utilized less frequently. The most widely used and generally available of these products is soyabean meal and this product is nutritionally attractive in poultry feed formulation because of its favourable amino acid pattern.

While vegetable protein materials are the most readily available, many of them contain anti-nutritive factors which must be removed by processing, for example heat treatment to remove the trypsin inhibitors in soyabean meal, or in some cases by plant breeding to produce genotypes in which these factors are reduced to acceptable levels, for example in oilseed rape (colza) where plant breeders have produced low glucosinolate and low erucic acid varieties which can be used in a wider range of feed formulations than the original cultivars.

Trypsin inhibitors are widely distributed in feed raw materials and are found in legumes such as soyabeans, peas and many species of beans. They are also found in some cereals such as rye, triticale and barley.

Extracted soyabean meal

Soyabeans are now the most widely grown oilseed in the world and are primarily produced for the high-quality oil they produce. Extracted soyabean meal is produced by solvent extraction of the meal to remove the oil and the resulting residual meal is then toasted to destroy the trypsin inhibitors present in the meal. The heat processing of soyabean meal requires a careful balance between applying sufficient heat to destroy the trypsin inhibitors but avoiding overheating that would cause denaturation of the protein.

Properly processed soyabean meal is one of the highest quality vegetable proteins available for poultry feeds. It is available either dehulled with the fibrous seed coats removed or with the hulls remaining in the product. While either product is suitable for feeding to older laying poultry, the dehulled product with its higher energy content is usually preferred for young birds such as broilers or turkey poults.

The trypsin inhibitors of raw soyabean cause depressed growth and pancreatic hypertrophy when fed to animals (Struthers and MacDonald 1983). They reduce protein digestibility by reducing the activity of proteolytic enzymes produced by the pancreas. In addition to reduced growth, due to poor protein digestion, poultry fed underprocessed soyabean meal produce wet droppings resulting in poor litter condition. This has been reported as a cause of pododermatitis—lesions of the sole of the foot—in broilers or turkeys (Jensen et al. 1970), which often then leads to carcase quality problems as a result of breast blisters or burned hocks.

Raw soyabeans also contain haemagglutinins or lectins which are thought to be partly responsible for the depression of feed conversion efficiency in the chick when underprocessed soyabean meals are fed.

Full-fat soyabeans

In recent years research workers and the feed industry have successfully explored the processing and use of whole soyabeans in livestock feeding, particularly in poultry production. The whole bean contains approximately 38% crude protein and about 18% oil. The advantages of using full-fat soya as an ingredient in poultry feeds are the high energy content resulting from the high level of very digestible oil in well-processed material and also the contribution of the essential fatty acid linoleic acid. Linoleic acid is essential for chick growth and is an important factor in feeding the commercial layer due to its positive effect in increasing egg weight (Han et al. 1988). Soyabean oil contains about 50% linoleic acid.

As is the case with extracted soyabean meal, full-fat soyabeans must be effectively heat treated to destroy the anti-nutritive factors associated with the whole bean. In addition the processing renders the fat contained in the bean accessible to digestion; methods of processing which disrupt the cell walls result in a product with higher fat digestibility and metabolizable energy content than alternative processes which are not so destructive. The mechanical shearing effects of extruder cookers have been shown to be very effective in this regard.

Extracted sunflower meal

Sunflowers are grown for oilseed production in many temperate and subtropi-

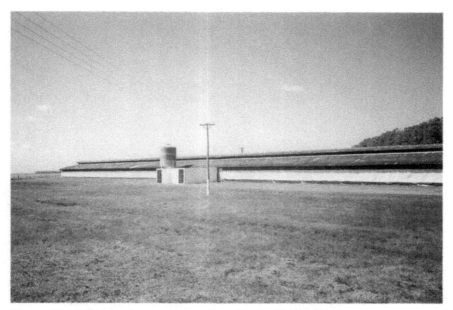

Plate 1 Typical broiler house with side curtains used in hotter climates.

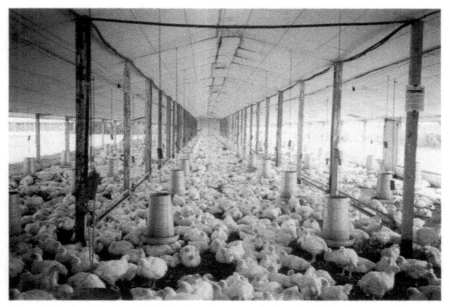

Plate 2 Broilers in open-sided housing (Argentina). Curtains have been raised.

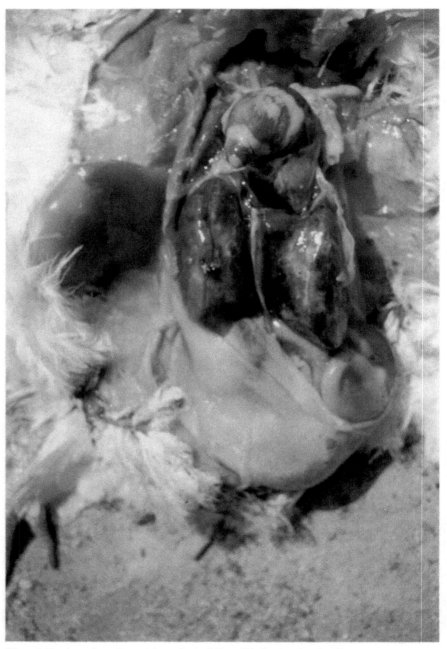

Plate 3 Lesion of perihepatitis typical of *E. coli* infection in a broiler.

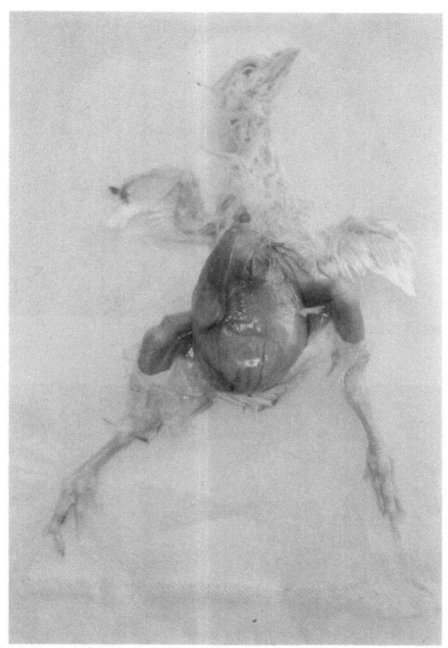

Plate 4 Yolk sac infection in a young chick.

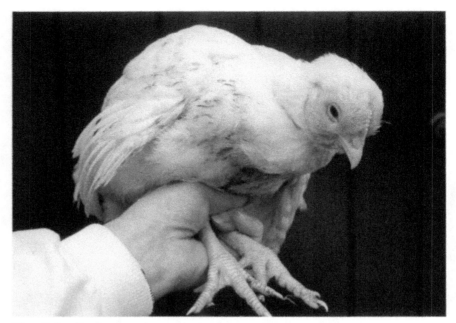

Plate 5 Swollen head syndrome in a broiler.

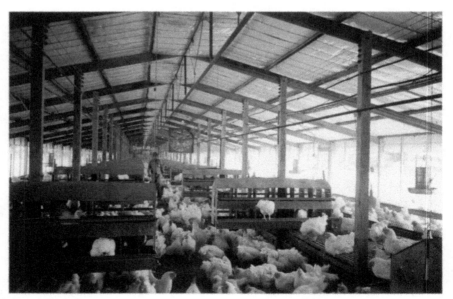

Plate 6 In many countries breeders are kept on a combination of litter and slats. Nest boxes are at right-angles to the slats. Note cockerel feeders (pan) and pullet feeders with grid.

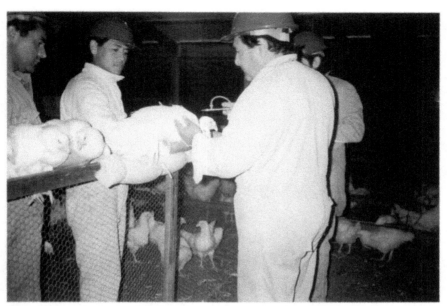

Plate 7 Administration of a killed vaccine by subcutaneous injection in the back of the neck.

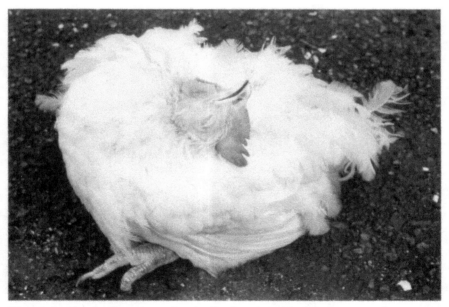

Plate 8 Swollen head syndrome in a broiler breeder with typical nervous signs.

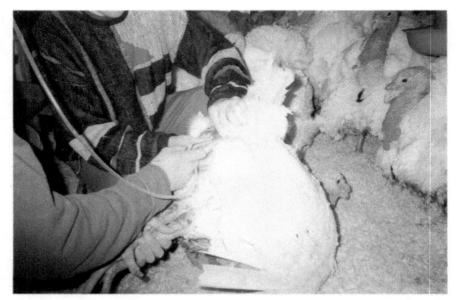

Plate 9 Artificial insemination—collection from the stag.

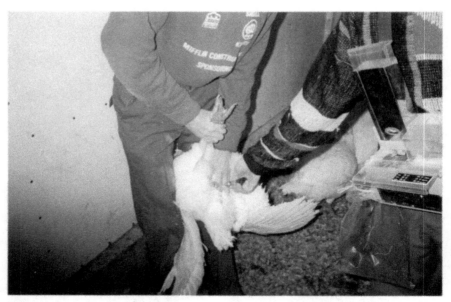

Plate 10 Insemination of the hen.

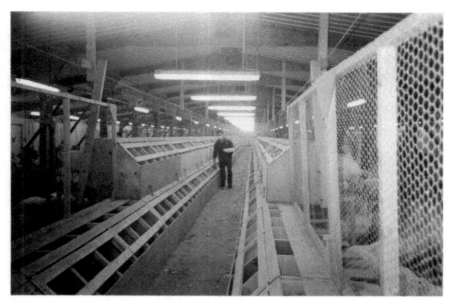

Plate 11 Nest boxes can be located either side of a central passageway to simplify egg collection.

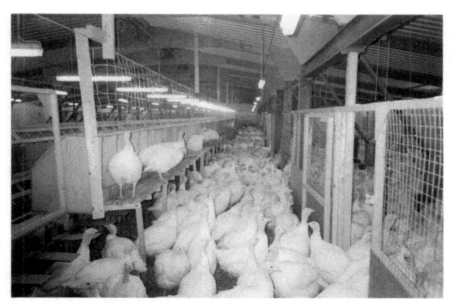

Plate 12 Female houses contain pens with gates so that birds can be kept away from nest boxes at night. This helps broody control.

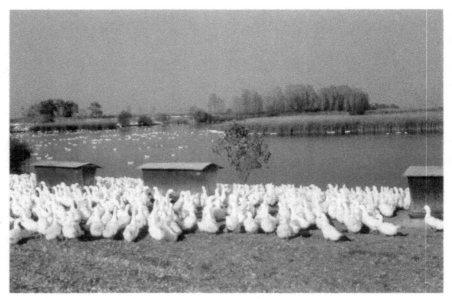

Plate 13 Growing ducklings on ponds (Hungary).

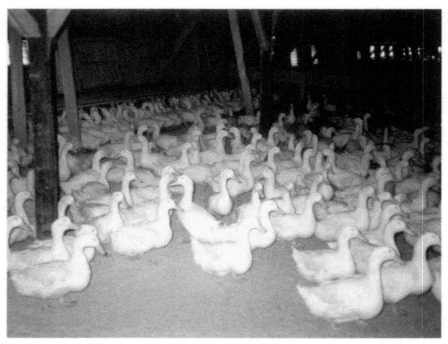

Plate 14 Young breeders on restricted feed and nipple drinkers (USA).

cal countries. Sunflower oil is a premium cooking oil which is high in polyunsaturated fatty acids. Sunflower meal is produced by solvent extraction; the meal may contain all the hulls, leaving a relatively high fibre content, or it may be partially dehulled, which produces a product higher in protein and energy and lower in fibre than the whole seed meal. The dehulled products are preferred for inclusion in poultry feeds. Sunflower oil is even higher in linoleic acid than is soya oil (at about 63% of the total oil content) and makes a useful contribution to the requirement of this essential fatty acid in chick or layer diets (Karunajeewa *et al.* 1989).

Sunflower meal is relatively free of anti-nutritional factors that may affect production.

Rapeseed meal

Oilseed rape is a crop of the genus *Brassica* grown in temperate climates. There are two species, *B. napus* and *B. campestris*. It has recently become very popular in Europe and Canada as a break crop in cereal rotations.

Rapeseed meal is available as either a high-oil expeller-processed product or a solvent-extracted meal. The solvent-extracted material is of higher quality than the expeller meal.

The protein content of rapeseed is of high quality but until relatively recently rapeseed meal was considered to be completely unsuitable for inclusion in poultry feeds due to its content of anti-nutritional factors. Rapeseed contains erucic acid and glucosinolates which, when hydrolysed by the enzyme myrosinase, produce isothionates. These isothionates affect the metabolism of iodine and the activity of the thyroid gland.

In recent years plant breeders in Canada and Europe have produced the so-called 'double zero' varieties of rapeseed in which the content of erucic acid and glucosinolate are reduced to very low levels and these are now finding a place in non-ruminant feeding. Double zero rapeseed meal is marketed in Canada under the brand name Canola Meal in order to distinguish this product from the high glucosinolate meals.

In addition to glucosinolates some varieties of rapeseed contain tannins which may affect growth rate in chickens or turkeys.

Problems of egg taint in eggs have been associated with the feeding of rapeseed to brown egg-laying strains of hens (Hobson-Frohock *et al.* 1973; Fenwick and Curtis 1980; Griffiths *et al.* 1979). The taint, which is variously described as fishy or musty, is due to trimethylamine which is derived from sinapine, a polyphenolic choline ester which is associated with the glucosinolate complex in rapeseed. This problem appears to be related to both high and low glucosinolate varieties of rapeseed, therefore it is generally accepted that rapeseed should not be fed to brown egg-laying strains of commercial layers.

A further problem which has been reported in connection with rapeseed meal is that of liver haemorrhage in laying hens and in broilers (Slominski *et al.* 1988). There appears to be a lower incidence of this problem with low-glucosinolate meals.

Animal proteins

Animal proteins include marine products manufactured from fish and products manufactured from offals and bones from abattoir and poultry processing.

Animal protein products provide readily available supplies of essential amino acids in feeds for non-ruminant animals including poultry. As the protein is derived from animal tissue it generally closely corresponds to the amino acid pattern required by the animal. In addition many of the products contain significant quantities of the major minerals calcium and phosphorus.

Fish meals

Fish meals are manufactured from either fish offal and skeletons derived from fish processing or from whole fish harvested specifically for fish meal production. Most of the fish offal meals are produced from white fish and have a relatively low oil content while most of the industrial fishing is for oily fishes such as herring, capelin, anchovy, pilchard and menhaden. By far the bulk of fish meal comes from industrial fishing.

Well-processed fish meal is an excellent source of protein for poultry with high levels of lysine and methionine of excellent biological availability and is free from the protease inhibitors which are present in many seed protein sources. It is also relatively high in energy in comparison with many sources of vegetation protein. In addition to this contribution of high-quality protein fish meal contains significant levels of calcium and readily available phosphorus.

The oil in fish meal is very unsaturated and contains high levels of long-chain unsaturated fatty acids. As a result the inclusion of fish meal in poultry feeds for both laying and table poultry must be limited in order to avoid egg or carcase taint. In order to prevent storage oxidation of the oil some manufacturers include an antioxidant in the meal. The advantage of this is that it maintains the level of energy of the fish meal but the disadvantge is that it also preserves the most highly unsaturated fatty acids which are associated with carcase taint and the development of 'off' flavours on storage of poultry meat products. The presence of trimethylammine in fish meals may also lead to taint in eggs from some brown egg-laying strains of commercial layers (Wakeling 1982).

In most cases fish meals are free from nutritional complications. However, there is one specific disease problem, gizzard erosion in broilers, which has been associated with some fish meals (Itakura *et al.* 1981). Research has shown that the overheating during processing of some fish meals containing high levels of histidine results in the production of a substance called gizzerosine, which has been shown to cause gizzard erosion (Masumara *et al.* 1985; Wessela and Post 1989).

Meat and bone meals

Meat and bone meals are produced from offals and butchery wastes, predominantly from the red meat industry although in some cases they may contain material from poultry processing factories. The composition of the products is somewhat variable depending on the source of material and protein levels can range from 40% to 60%, oil levels from 1% to 15% and ash levels from 20% to 40% depending on the raw material and whether or not the oil or tallow is solvent extracted or mechanically separated. The calcium and phosphorus levels in the product are in direct relation to the level of ash, which in turn is dependent on the amount of bone in the raw material processed. The product is generally free from anti-nutritional factors although occasional problems have been reported from time to time of high chromium levels resulting from the inclusion of tannery waste in the raw material.

Poultry processing by-products

The by-products of poultry processing are used in the manufacture of feather meal, poultry offal meal or a combined feather and offal meal. While the processes used in the manufacture of these products are capable of efficiently sterilizing them there is always the danger of post-processing contamination with pathogenic organisms from raw material within the processing plant.

The processing of feathers to produce feather meal entails their hydrolysis by cooking with steam under pressure in order to improve the digestibility of the protein. The protein of feather meal is poorly utilized by poultry (Bielorai *et al.* 1982).

Poultry offal meal is manufactured by cooking the offal and other parts of the carcase which are not required for human consumption. Products from poultry processing plants involved in further processing will contain larger amounts of bone, due to the inclusion of quantities of stripped carcases, and will therefore have higher mineral contents. During the process poultry oil is separated from the meal but the latter still contains a relatively high level of oil. The product is a good source of both amino acids and energy when it is well processed in a hygienically well-controlled manufacturing plant (Escalona and Pesti 1987).

Mixed poultry offal and feather meal is a lower grade material due to the compromise in conditions required to process the different components of the product and its content of the nutritionally inferior feather meal.

Moulds and mycotoxins

Feed raw materials, particularly those field crops such as cereals which are incorporated in the feed with a minimum of processing, usually carry considerable numbers of fungal spores. Poultry production problems caused by fungi fall into three main categories:

1. A direct mycotic infection in the bird, e.g. aspergillosis, a mycosis caused by *Aspergillus fumigatus*.
2. Changes in the nutritional composition of the feed as a result of the growth of the mould by destruction of vitamins or reduction in energy level of the feed.
3. The production of mycotoxins.

Mycotoxins are secondary metabolites produced by fungi and are present in the feed prior to it being fed to the bird. A feed ingredient may be infected by the fungus in the field due to crop damage resulting from adverse climatic conditions or insect infestation, but raw materials can be affected by moulds leading to the development of mycotoxins, as the result of poor storage at high moisture levels, either in the feed mill or on the farm. Finished feeds can also develop moulds and mycotoxins, particularly when stored in moist warm conditions with poor ventilation.

Problems with mycotoxins have been recognized and experienced for many years. Probably the best known of these was ergot (*Claviceps purpurea*), which classically affects rye and triticale but also is relatively common in wheat. However, the appearance of turkey X disease in 1960 in Great Britain and the subsequent identification of a link between the disease and aflatoxin from Brazilian groundnut meal stimulated substantial research into mycotoxins and established their significance in animal disease. Since that time over 200 mycotoxins have been identified. Of these aflatoxin, ochratoxin, the trichothene toxins including T-2 and vomitoxin and zearalenone are regarded as the most significant in livestock production.

Many of the problems of mycotoxins at low, chronic levels are difficult to diagnose specifically and are expressed only as apparently non-specific depression in performance that is unaccountable to any other cause.

Aflatoxin

Aflatoxin is the most widespread of the mycotoxins and is produced by *Aspergillus flavus* or *A. parasiticus*. It has been reported on a wide variety of products including groundnuts, cottonseed, copra, palm kernels, maize, sorghum, wheat, barley and rye. Sixteen aflatoxins have been identified of which four naturally occurring ones, aflatoxins B1, B2, G1 and G2, are highly toxic. Aflatoxin affects growth in poultry at very low levels, with as little as 100 ppb (0.1 mg/kg) producing significantly depressed growth in ducklings or turkey poults (Howell 1982). The most susceptible poultry are ducklings followed by turkeys, goslings and chickens, with adult laying hens the least susceptible (Arafa *et al.* 1981). The level of aflatoxin required to depress egg production in layers is less than 2.5 ppm. The signs of aflatoxicosis at very low concentrations of the mycotoxin are non-specific—reductions in growth rate and deterioration of feed conversion rate for no other apparent reason are the most common observations. The mycotoxin also results in impaired immunity to disease. On post-mortem the liver is enlarged with fatty infiltration and at larger doses the pancreas, spleen and bursa of Fabricius are also enlarged. Economic losses include not only those resulting from decreased growth performance but also there is increased susceptibility to carcase bruising leading to downgrading (Tung *et al.* 1971).

EC countries have statutory controls on the maximum amount of aflatoxin permitted in straight feedstuffs for livestock including poultry, and in compound feedstuffs. These limits as enacted in UK legislation are shown in Table 4.10.

Table 4.10 Maximum contents of aflatoxin permitted in feedingstuffs for poultry under Feedingstuffs Regulations (1991) in the UK (Source: HMSO SI 1991 No. 2480)

Feedingstuff	Maximum content of Aflatoxin mg/kg
Straight feedingstuffs except	0.05
groundnut, copra, palm-kernel, cotton seed, babassu, maize	
and products derived from the processing thereof	0.02
Complete feedingstuffs for pigs and poultry (except piglets and chicks)	0.02
Other complete feedingstuffs	0.01
Complementary feedingstuffs for pigs and poultry (except young	
animals)	0.03
Other complementary feedingstuffs	0.005

Ochratoxin

The main toxic component of the ochratoxin complex of mycotoxins is ochra-toxin-A. This can be produced by a number of widespread *Aspergillus* and *Penicillium* species some of which can also produce the mycotoxin citrinin. It normally occurs in temperate climates, and in a UK survey Buckle (1981) found about 19.6% of samples of barley and 14.7% of samples of wheat examined between 1976 and 1979 to contain this mycotoxin.

Ochratoxin is highly toxic to chickens, inhibiting growth at a dietary level as low as 1 ppm. Layers show decreased egg production at 500 ppb and decreased egg size at 1 ppm of ochratoxin (Howell 1982). Even lower concentrations cause diarrhoea in layers, resulting in an increase in numbers of soiled and stained eggs. Ochratoxin is nephrotoxic and causes decreased bone strength in young broilers. Pathological changes include proventricular haemorrhages and visceral gout. Ochratoxin A causes increased blood clotting time and increased susceptibility to bruising.

Trichothecenes

The trichothecenes are a large group of mycotoxins produced by *Fusarium* species. The most important for poultry are the T-2 toxin produced by *F. tricinctum*, and vomitoxin (deoxynivalenol) produced by *F. graminarum*. The characteristic signs of T-2 toxicosis in broiler chickens are necrotic oral lesions and neural lesions leading to nervous seizures. The toxin also causes abnormal feathering in chickens with feathers protruding at unusual angles, and also leads to reduced weight gains (Hoerr *et al.* 1982a). Reduced resistance to salmonellosis in chickens has been associated with T-2 toxin. Laying hens exhibit oral lesions, reduced feed consumption, lowered egg production and thinner egg shells when fed 20 ppm of the toxin (Wyatt *et al.* 1975). All these factors would have a serious effect on the economic returns from the flock.

Zearalenone

This mycotoxin occurs very frequently in the USA where it is commonly associated with mouldy corn. Zearalenone (F-2 toxin) is produced by a range of *Fusarium* species and can occur in cereal grain crops in the UK (Hacking *et al.* 1976). The toxin causes problems at levels as low as 500 ppb (0.5 mg/kg). It is oestrogenic in its activity and has caused reproductive problems in farm livestock, particularly in pigs. Signs in poultry are less obvious than in the mammalian livestock species, although reduced growth rates and swollen vents have been recorded in turkeys. In laying hens feed intake is depressed and egg production reduced with some reports of hens ceasing to lay.

The mycotoxins are clearly very toxic. However, they are generally only associated with vegetable raw materials which are subject to fungal spoilage at harvesting or during storage. Poor standards of storage and handling of finished feeds, even up to the point of feeding in the poultry house, can result in accumulation of stale feed and encourage mould growth and the production of mycotoxins. Good feed hygiene is extremely important and the need to clean storage bins and silos and feeding equipment cannot be overemphasized. Feeders in poultry houses should be correctly adjusted to avoid spillage. Mould inhibitors based on organic acids such as propionic acid can be used to reduce fungal contamination of feed. Pelleting of feed can also be an advantage. It has been shown that pelleting can reduce mould counts by a factor of 100 to 10 000 depending on the sample (Tabib *et al.* 1984).

Quality control

The quality control of feeds used in poultry production plays an essential part in ensuring the quality of the finished poultry products. Only by careful control at all stages in the manufacture of feeds from the earliest stages of ingredient specification through to the checking of the finished feed to ensure that it complies with the intentions of the nutritionist can the performance be ensured.

Quality control of raw materials

There are a number of potential pitfalls which can occur between the specification and formulation of feeds and their ultimate presentation to the animal. The quality control of feeds commences at the earliest stages of procurement of the feed ingredients. Questions which may arise in relation to the control of feed ingredient supplies cover such areas as:

1. Do the raw materials received from suppliers correspond to the buying specification agreed with them when the purchase was made?
2. Do the nutritional data ascribed to the raw material in formulating the feed correspond to the actual analysis of the materials received from the supplier and used in manufacture?
3. Are the raw materials actually received and used in manufacture consistent in analysis from batch to batch?
4. If in the course of manufacture of a raw material, a process is applied in

order to remove or reduce the level of an inherent anti-nutritional factor, is this process effectively carried out and is the raw material received consistently within the specific limits for the factor involved?

In order to control the quality of raw materials entering the production process it is important that a system of approval of raw materials and sources of supply is established. Such an approval system can be formalized to provide a sound framework for both nutritionists and buyers, and is described below.

Before any purchase of an ingredient the buyer should agree a specification with the supplier. The buyer must therefore obtain from the potential supplier sufficiently detailed information to allow the particular source of the material to be assessed and compared with characteristics for the ingredient in question. In the case of commonly used products there is a wealth of data with which this information can be compared. It cannot be assumed that ingredients from different sources having the same name and broad description are identical, due to differences in source of raw material and in the manufacturing process where this is relevant. The data obtained from the supplier should be assessed by the feed formulator in conjunction with the buyer in order that the ingredient source can be compared with any other sources of similar material currently being used, so enabling an assessment of whether or not the new source can be effectively substituted for the existing materials. Wherever possible the quality control manager should visit the manufacturing plant where the material is produced in order to obtain a sound understanding of the problems of the production process and the levels of management and control in the manufacture of the potential raw material source. If the product at this juncture appears satisfactory the procurement process can move to the next stage.

Wherever possible it is sound procedure for the supplier to provide a number of samples of the product over a period of time from the normal production run for investigation in order that these may be assessed against the information obtained from the supplier. Analysis of these samples should be carried out by a competent laboratory and cover all critical aspects of the raw material in relation to its specific nutrient contribution to the end feed product and any potential problems associated with the material. The results of analysis of these samples will provide some information on the degree of variability of the product from batch to batch.

At this stage any problems which have been revealed should be discussed with the supplier with a view to their resolution if this is possible.

If on reviewing the information accumulated on the material it still meets the technical requirements, the process of procurement can be extended to the purchase of trial commercial quantities over a defined period of time. During this period the product remains under relatively intensive analytical scrutiny. Any practical logistical problems of supply, with any handling and manufacturing problems will also be revealed as these inevitably will create quality problems for the end feed product, should they occur. During this period of trial supply the data should be kept under constant review by both nutritionists and buyers pending a final decision on whether or not the material or source of supply should be approved for general use. At this stage a finalized formal specification can be drawn up for the raw material from the specific source. This should be agreed with the seller and form part of the purchase contract.

Routine quality control of approved raw materials should start at the reception of the ingredient into the mill. Each consignment should be examined to see that it is typical of the product in appearance and smell. It should be free from any signs of spoilage such as evidence of mould. Samples of the product should be taken regularly for laboratory analysis. The assays carried out by the laboratory should be chosen with reference to the specification of the product and should pay due regard to the specific characteristics and critical aspects of the raw material's composition, particularly to those factors which are affected in the production processes of the raw material. For example in the production of extracted dehulled soya meal the processing involves the removal of the hulls, the solvent extraction of the oil and the inactivation of trypsin inhibitors in the residual meal and the stripping of residual solvent from the meal by steam. The purchase contract will also probably specify the minimum protein content of the product. The laboratory quality control (QC) profile for extracted dehulled soya meal should therefore include assays for moisture, crude protein, ether extract, crude fibre and trypsin inhibition.

Routine quality control reports should be reviewed critically on a regular basis and any deficiencies against specification must be communicated to the buyer, who should then inform the product supplier. If the quality control procedure reveals regular problems with a product then serious consideration should be given to discontinuing supplies from that source.

While some information can be obtained from the results of individual samples, it is a good plan to maintain a running sequential record of analytical results. This enables assessment of any trends in the characteristics of the raw material and provides a good basis for the formulator to take decisions on any adjustments to the raw material database which may be necessary. Additionally, if sufficient samples are analysed within a given period of delivery, they can be statistically analysed for standard deviation and a good objective measurement of variability of the product can be obtained.

Quality control of finished feeds

Provided there is an effective system of quality control of raw materials, quality control of the finished feed is relatively simple and only relates to assessing the efficiency of its manufacture.

The objective of the QC procedure is to ensure that the formulation objectives in terms of the supply of nutrients are properly translated and that the intended levels of these nutrients are achieved in the end-product. As in the case of raw material, quality control attention must be focused on identifiable critical areas where problems may occur in the manufacturing process. It is also important that account is taken of aspects of the feed which may be critical to the performance of the birds or the quality of the end-product.

Questions arising in routine quality control of finished poultry feeds are listed below:

1. Does the feed proximate analysis for the major constituents protein, oil and ash correspond with the calculated analysis of these aspects of the product?
2. Major mineral levels can be critical in poultry feeds. Is the sodium chloride level within acceptable limits? (Excess salt levels can cause wet litter and resulting foot and carcase quality problems in table poultry and egg soiling problems in commercial egg layers or breeders. The margin of error in adding these to the feed mix is relatively small.) Is the calcium level in the layer or breeder feed at the correct level? (Deficiencies in calcium will lead to shell quality problems and consequent downgrading which can lead to substantial loss in revenue in layer flocks.)
3. Is any supplement containing trace minerals and vitamins (and perhaps prophylactic medicines such as coccidiostats or histomonostats) included at the correct level? (If not the recipient birds may suffer specific nutrient deficiencies or may not be adequately protected against parasitic diseases leading to poor performance or mortality.)
4. In cases where premixes of medicinal substances are added independently of nutritional supplements are they being added accurately?

As in the case of quality control of feed ingredients a formal regime of sampling should be instituted with a predetermined profile of analysis for feeds intended for different classes of poultry. All laboratory samples of poultry feed should be assayed for protein, oil and ash. They should also be assayed for a trace mineral as an indicator of the presence of the feed supplement. In the case of poultry feeds manganese is a good choice as its assay is relatively straightforward and it is normally added routinely to poultry feeds.

In addition sufficient feed samples for table poultry, including broilers, turkeys and ducks, should be analysed for salt and assayed for any medicinal substances to ensure that they are being added at the correct level and are adequately distributed in the feed. In the case of feeds for laying and breeding poultry regular assays for calcium should also be carried out.

The basic approach for the interpretation of finished feed analysis results is essentially similar to that described for raw materials with data both on an individual sample and a more global basis assisting in the interpretation of the efficiency of the manufacturing process. It is extremely important that assay results should be seen by the quality control and production management on a regular basis and action taken promptly where problems are exposed. Assay results which remain confined to the laboratory notebook are of no value in quality control.

While the catalogue of health problems described in this chapter must appear somewhat daunting and give the impression that feed is a major health hazard in poultry production, almost all the problems described can be avoided by sound specification and formulation of the feed, judicious choice of raw materials and efficient quality control.

Further reading

Nixey C, Grey T C (eds) (1989) *Recent advances in turkey science.* Butterworths, London.
Scott M L, Neisheim M C, Young R J (1976) *Nutrition of the chicken.* M L Scott & Associates, New York.
Wiseman J (ed) (1987) *Feeding of non ruminant livestock.* Butterworths, London.

5 DISEASE PREVENTION AND CONTROL IN BROILERS

MARK A. GOODWIN DVM, MAM, PhD, Dipl.
ACPV, JOHN BROWN DVM, PhD, LUCY M.
ROWLAND MS, MLS

Introduction

Disease prevention in any flock involves the shared responsibility of many persons, adherence to industry standards, and a team approach to production. To assure disease prevention and control, poultry producers must maintain records of health performance and subscribe to good management practices. All members of the production team should clearly understand both their own role and that of others in growing and maintaining healthy poultry. To foster this, management must train individuals not only in their own production tasks but also in the tasks of their co-workers. This education process should be on-going to ensure that workers remain abreast of new developments. It has been said that the quality of communications can have as much impact on productivity as any other production or management variable.

Principal aspects of management and disease prevention

Good management is essential to disease prevention and control in broilers. This involves selection of high-quality chicks followed by a good programme of disease prevention including routine vaccination, good environmental control, sanitary housing and modern equipment that is well maintained.

Attention to the details involved with the management and control of the environment and nutrition of the chicks will ultimately produce the highest profits.

Prevention of disease

About 96% of the broilers started in the poultry-producing areas of the USA reach market weight and are sold for human consumption. Most of the remaining chicks succumb to disease, with an estimated 80–90% of these lost as a result of management failures. The production programme must emphasize a good disease prevention strategy to minimize losses. Disease prevention through sound management will be more profitable than poor management that relies on vaccinations and medications to deal with health problems.

Biosecurity

The single best disease prevention technique is to avoid exposing chicks to disease (see Chapter 2). Healthy, properly nourished chicks that are housed in a sanitary well-ventilated and well-controlled environment will remain healthy if other good management practices are also observed.

Poultry workers and equipment are two major sources of pathogenic agents for broilers. Therefore biosecurity is a critical management tool that involves all workers who come in contact with the flock at all stages of production. Biosecurity should be included in training programmes for *all* people who are in contact with the birds.

A biosecurity programme is based on allowing the birds to come into contact only with personnel who are essential to the poultry house operation. Access to the farm and its houses should be denied except to those actively responsible for the welfare of the poultry. Visitors simply should not be allowed; signs posted on the premises should state this policy and help with enforcement. While sophisticated electronic gate security systems are available, a simple padlock, key and chain system is sufficient. To enter the farm or poultry house, workers should wear disinfected boots, or sturdy disposable boots, single-use overalls and a hat.

The farm manager should maintain a cleansing (soap and water) wash-down station and require hosing down of service vehicles that enter the farm. Such vehicles always should be clean inside and outside. No debris or dirt should be present. Furthermore, the floor mats and operating pedals should be sprayed with disinfectant each time the operator leaves a farm.

Relaxing biosecurity programmes may save money in the short term, but any consequent entry of disease will increase costs and may cause financial losses in either the short or long term.

Chick quality

To ensure the uniform quality of the broiler flock, selected chicks should have the following characteristics:

1. Healthy parents. This means that the breeding flock should be free of infectious disease agents, including *Mycoplasma gallisepticum*, *M. synoviae*, and *Salmonella pullorum*, as well as genetic diseases or defects.
2. Uniform size and colour.
3. Clean, dry and fluffy appearance. Healthy chicks will have closed, healed navels, clean vents and the unfeathered skin over the legs will be bright and smooth.
4. Bright, alert and active. They should be free of congenital deformities.

Chicks originating from a single breeder flock should be used to fill a house whenever possible. This strategy promotes uniformity within the finished broiler flock. One age/one site or all in/all out flock management makes vaccination, sanitation and nutrition easier to manage.

Good breeder and hatchery management is essential to the production of quality eggs and quality chicks (see Chapter 3). It is estimated that good quality hatching eggs result in 2% more saleable chicks. For broiler producers, this probably is manifest by a 2% increase in liveability.

Chick placement and brooding density

Newly hatched chicks have yolks which store about 2 g of fat and 2.5 ml of water. The energy content of the fat will meet all energy requirements of the chick for about 2–3 days. The water store will last from 8 hours to 2 days, depending upon ambient environmental temperature. Optimal preparation of the broiler chick's environment, food and water are crucial if the chick is to survive and thrive.

Before new chicks arrive, the broiler house and its equipment should be thoroughy cleaned of organic matter as described in Chapter 2.

The housing environment must be stabilized prior to the arrival of the chicks. This environmental regulation includes proper temperature, humidity, ventilation, and lights. Fresh feed and water should be in place before the chicks are introduced. Constant access to clean water is important: chicks that do not drink will not eat, and will succumb quickly. Prior to the arrival of the chicks the water line and all individual watering devices should be filled. The watering devices should be tested to ensure they deliver water adequately and do not leak.

Feed lines should always be emptied of finishing ration and should be cleaned and disinfected between each depopulation. Additionally, all feed containers must be dry prior to filling in order to prevent bacterial or fungal spoilage of the ration.

Each brooder should be operating normally. The house air temperature should be stabilized at 31 °C (95 °F) (see page 147). The ventilation fans should be operating and providing good air movement without draughts (see Chapter 2).

Healthy chicks should be transported to the farm in well-ventilated chick buses. Poor ventilation will result in oxygen-deprived and overheated chicks, and weakness or failure to eat or drink will follow. In more extreme cases, death results from suffocation.

If air circulation in a bus full of chicks stops, the air temperature will increase at 0.8 °C (1.5 °F) per minute. At this rate, the air temperature in chick trays in a stationary bus can rapidly climb to some 14 °C (25 °F) higher than the outside air temperature. Chicks kept at temperatures of over 37.7 °C (100 °F) are oxygen-deprived and heat-stressed.

Boxes of chicks should be unloaded outside and carried into the house; there is a potential health hazard to both humans and chicks from carbon monoxide poisoning if buses are driven into the house. To eliminate this risk, bus engines always should be shut off while unloading the chicks.

To ensure adequate ventilation when chicks are unloaded, boxes should not be stacked over three high. Great care should be exercised in removing chicks from the boxes to prevent injury. This means that when lifting the chicks out of the box they should slowly tumble and not fall.

The disposable chick pads should be destroyed or otherwise disposed of on the farm. Plastic chick boxes can be re-used after returning to the hatchery for final washing and sanitation.

Trouble-shooting common maladies of young chicks generally is not difficult:

New arrivals:
- Chicks gasp. This is either caused by fumigation with formaldehyde at the hatchery, or infection with *Aspergillus* spp. or other fungi.
- Chicks pant and are lethargic. This probably indicates overheating during transport. Make sure the chicks drink water within one hour of placement.
- Chicks are uncoordinated, have laboured breathing. This is due to oxygen deficit during and immediately after hatching.

First week:
- Chicks sit, huddle, are reluctant to feed or drink. This is probably due

to chilling during transit. Increase brooding temperature about 1 °C and move the food and water closer to the chicks.

- Immediate, high mortality. Other chicks are weak, huddle together, and many have watery droppings. If the umbilical area appears infected or the abdomen is soft and large, then there is omphalitis. The hatchery should be notified. Increase brooding temperature. Although these chicks can be treated with antibiotics, such treatment usually is not efficacious and, therefore, is not recommended.
- Chicks are agitated, weak. Legs may appear dry and spindly. Chicks probably are dehydrated. Increase drinker space by 50% for 24 hours. Add vitamins and electrolytes to the water.
- High mortality, days 3–5.
  - Chicks are emaciated, have never eaten ('starve-outs'). May be caused by over- or under-heating. Check and adjust brooding temperature.
  - Chicks have faecal material pasted around vent area. The usual cause is overheating. Check and adjust brooding temperature.
  - Chicks have difficulty walking, appear sore. Usually due to eggs that are incubated and hatched upside-down.

Disinfectants

Sanitizers, disinfectants and sterilizing compounds can be a valuable part of a sound custodial programme that limits the growing chickens' exposure to pathogenic organisms. However, there is no substitute for cleanliness and neatness.

Thorough cleaning is probably more beneficial than the application of a disinfectant on a marginally dirty surface. Application of disinfectant to a dirty surface does not kill all pathogens and therefore usually wastes time and money, and places the health of chicks at risk. To safeguard the health of chickens, a thorough cleaning followed by a disinfectant on a clean surface is the best strategy.

Disinfectants are very effective if they are used properly. Compounds such as the coal-tar distillates, synthetic phenols, and quaternary ammonium compounds are not susceptible to inactivation by small amounts of organic material, and as a result are well suited for use in poultry houses. However, even within these groups some compounds and formulations are more effective than others, especially when organic material is present. Therefore, thorough cleaning before disinfection will make the disinfection procedure more efficacious.

Whichever disinfectant is chosen, it is absolutely necessary to read and follow the manufacturer's directions for use. For example, some soaps and disinfectants are incompatible. Non-ionic soaps should be used with quaternary ammonia compounds and phenols. Chlorine inactivates quaternary ammonia compounds and phenols upon direct contact. Usually, disinfectants are applied by spraying or foaming with a medium pressure sprayer. After disinfection, allow the house and equipment to dry completely.

Feeders, hoppers and feed bins should be scraped and scrubbed to remove old feed. When the old feed is removed completely, the bin should be washed with a 10% commercial bleach solution via a high-pressure sprayer. Flush out water lines and clean and disinfect all fixtures: waterers, tanks, proportioners and medicators.

It is an important part of the overall strategy to periodically use a different disinfectant. The use of several disinfectants on a rotational basis will prevent microorganisms from building up resistance to any one particular disinfectant.

Stocking density, brooding and growing

The objective of a housing system and the manner in which it is stocked with chicks is to maximize productivity and profitability, not simply to provide shelter for the birds.

Stocking density

Several variables enter into stocking density. These include:

1. Expected size of bird at market age;
2. Type of housing;
3. Cost of feed;
4. Time of year;
5. Market price.

The variables all relate to production costs and resulting profit margins.

Determining stocking density is a complex management issue. First, the expected size of the bird at the market age is relatively straightforward. Smaller size birds will permit a larger stocking density and vice versa. A sound management principle is that stocking density is determined by the expected market weight of the birds. In the USA a recommended standard is 29.3 kg market weight birds per m^2 (6 lb per ft^2). In the UK 34 kg/m^2 (7 lb/ft^2) is the maximum recommended by welfare codes. However, when the market for poultry is good, poultry producers overstock, and therefore overcrowd the flock. The overcrowding has several undesirable results, most notably the increased stress on the birds because of the reduced availability of feed and water and aggression between individuals. Additionally, stress suppresses the immune system and birds are much less capable of withstanding infections and surviving disease outbreaks. While, generally speaking, allotted floor space is dependent on the type of house construction (Table 5.1), exceeding the maximum recommended stocking density will have multiple adverse effects on poultry production.

Table 5.1 Broiler stocking density in relation to the type of house construction (USA guidelines)*

House construction	Stocking density	
	Birds/m^2	Birds/ft^2
Not insulated		
Spring, autumn, winter	10.8–13.5	0.8–1.0
Summer	9.0–10.8	1.0–1.2
Insulated	12.0	0.9
Controlled environment	13.5	0.8

* In the UK the maximum density recommended by welfare bodies is 34 kg/m^2 (7 lb/ft^2) market weight birds.

The cost of feed is a major factor in poultry production. When feed costs are low and the price of poultry is favourable, there is a tendency to increase production by increasing stocking density, leading to stress on the chickens in the flock and some losses.

Brooding and growing

Most experts assert that over 70% of the energy requirements for raising poultry are used in the brooding phase. This is the most critical time in the life of a market chicken, and the conditions to which birds are subjected during this time period are important both to the size and health of the finished broilers and to profits. The health of the bird at 59 days of age correlates with that of the bird from day 1 to day 14. Therefore, maintaining high production standards during the brooding phase will result in a better finished product that will sharply contrast with birds managed under suboptimal conditions. When energy or fuel is expensive there is usually a tendency to economize by providing less heat and inadequate ventilation at the time when it is needed most. This should be avoided as an inferior product will result.

Unlike older birds, newly hatched chicks have no means of regulating their body temperature. Therefore, young birds are totally dependent upon external environmental control for their comfort and survival. At about 21 days, the chick gradually begins to develop the capacity to regulate its own body temperature. Therefore, an essential element of brooding is temperature regulation using heat and circulating fresh air. Failure to provide proper ventilation *and* heating will result in either chilling or overheating, which in turn cause stress, starvation and dehydration, or in extreme cases, death of the birds.

Record keeping of environmental parameters is essential and should begin two days prior to the chicks being placed in the house for brooding. At least three times a day the brooding house temperature should be measured and plotted on a chart. Prior to checking temperatures the thermometers themselves should be cleaned so that they may be accurately read. Additionally, the thermometers should be checked for accuracy. The chicks should be observed at least three times a day for signs of discomfort. For example, sounds of distressed peeping and signs of huddling and clustering will indicate that they are either too hot or too cold. Recommended temperatures for growing broilers are listed in Table 5.2. Even though floor temperatures are higher, at 1.5 m (5 ft) above the litter, the temperature should be kept at 21.1 °C (70 °F). In the event of stress or reaction to vaccines, the floor temperature should be increased 2.8 °C (5 °F) above the recommended temperature until the birds return to normal.

Table 5.2 Environmental temperatures for maintenance of broilers, measured at 5 cm (2 in) above the litter

Age (days)	°C	°F
1–7	35	95
8–14	32.2	90
15–21	29.4	85
22–28	26.6	80
29–35	23.9	75
36–market	21.1	70

Manufacturers of brooding equipment make specific recommendations pertinent to the performance of their particular brooder. Given that the chicks are closely monitored for signs of discomfort, the manufacturer's recommendations should be followed closely. Again, use clean, dry litter for brooding. Damp litter absorbs heat, which otherwise should be used to warm the chicks.

Water is an important element of heat regulation and excretion, so an ample supply of clean water is essential to the brooding phase (Tables 5.3 and 5.4). It

Table 5.3 Typical water consumption of broilers

Age (weeks)	1	2	3	4	5	6	7	8
Litres consumed (per 1000 birds per hour)	19	57	94	132	169	203	241	278
Gallons	5	15	25	35	45	54	64	74

Table 5.4 Drinking space provision for broiler chicks

Watering system	Space
Trough/bell	2 cm (0.75 in)/chick
Fountain/cone/cup	1 waterer/100 birds
Nipple drinker	1/12–15 chicks

is important to note that when chicks fail to drink they also fail to eat, retarding growth and weight gain and making them more susceptible to disease. The end result is less poultry to market. It has been estimated that a 10% restriction of water consumption will cost a 40 000 chick broiler farm about $US2400 (1992 figures).

Birds should not have to travel in excess of 2.5 m (8 ft) to drink water. The water system should be inspected at least daily and kept clean. It is important that waterers be maintained at the correct height. The height of an open watering system (e.g. troughs) can be easily estimated as the point between the line parallel to the chicken's back and the line parallel to the chicken's eye. This means that chickens are not required to bend down in order to drink and will permit birds to consume water without spilling it. Closed systems (e.g. nipple drinkers) should be on a line level with the chicken's eye. It is important to adjust the height of the waterers gradually as birds grow. Adjust every other day for 2 weeks, then every day from that time on to market. After about 5 days, chicks on nipple drinker systems should have to reach up and stretch slightly to activate the nipple.

For the nipple drinkers to work, poultry-house floors must be level. Air leaks also can be a serious problem. Raising the pressure regulator end of the line slightly prevents air from getting down the line, and allows air to escape. Make sure that each nipple is receiving water and is operating properly.

Proper feeding is also essential to the brooding phase. Some general guidelines for food space availability are made in Table 5.5. Height is also important

Table 5.5 Feeding space provision for broiler chicks

Age (days)	Feeding space per chick
1–14	2.5 cm (1 in)
15–42	4.5 cm (1.75 in)
43–market	7.5 cm (3 in)

for feeders. As birds go through the starter, grower and finishing rations, the lip of the feeder pan should be level with the back of the bird. Feeders should be kept a third to half full but no more so as to avoid waste. As with the waterers, following the manufacturer's instructions is essential. The general goal is the lowest cost formulation that is consistent with minimum recommended feed standards, yet one generally nutritious enough to attain growth goals. However, much of a disease prevention programme is based not on a merely adequate diet, but on an optimal diet. Both nutritional deficiencies and excesses, and nutrient imbalances will cause disease and/or failure to thrive.

Nutritionally inadequate diets impair the immune system. When this occurs, chickens become susceptible to infectious diseases. A drop in feed consumption can be due to an increase in temperature, a decrease in water consumption or the onset of disease.

Vaccination requirements and methods

The vaccination programme

It is important to remember that a good vaccination programme is part of, but not a substitute for, good management. All major broiler-producing companies maintain their own policies and programmes regarding vaccinations. Within these programmes there are individual geographical variations, and problems unique to certain farms. In parallel with vaccination programmes are methods of objective disease diagnosis, and routine monitoring of both antibody levels and disease outbreaks. Proper management and interpretation of health records can provide information that will influence vaccination programmes, therefore a simple, readily understandable record form or system should always be employed.

Any tendency to change programmes based upon rumours, hunches or hearsay is not advisable as programmes of this type stand a good chance of failing—with expensive results.

Vaccination is *not* disease prevention. The purpose of vaccination is to enable a chicken to resist an infectious disease should it be infected.

A glaring failure in vaccination programmes reflects failure of communication among production managers, diagnosticians and poultry researchers. When vital information is compartmentalized, the success of the entire disease prevention programme is jeopardized.

Specific recommendations regarding a vaccination programme hinge on several factors, especially on the prevalence of each disease in the particular geographical area, and on the level of maternal antibodies.

Some diseases like Marek's disease, Newcastle disease, infectious bronchitis and avian encephalomyelitis are so prevalent world-wide and so easily and rapidly spread that it is almost impossible to avoid them. Therefore, vaccinating chicks at the appropriate age is the best way to avoid an outbreak. However, successful vaccination *will not* prevent infection, but it will prevent the manifestations of clinical disease in a healthy bird.

Disease is multifactorial involving the pathogenic agent, the host and the environment. For example, well-nourished chickens properly vaccinated with infectious bronchitis (IB) disease virus, maintained in a well-ventilated ammonia-free house will not become diseased when infected with the virus. On the other hand, a failure in ventilation or nutrition will place even properly vaccinated birds with demonstrable IB antibody at risk due to stress.

There are three general philosophies regarding timing of vaccination as an adjunct to preventing disease. Firstly, high levels of antibodies are produced by immunizing the hens. Chicks therefore will receive high levels of maternal antibodies from the hen through the yolk (passive immunity), and as a result the chick vaccination programme would be minimal. Secondly, if breeder antibody levels are low, chicks must be vaccinated in order to achieve the proper level of antibodies (active acquired immunity). Lastly, the newest concept is *in ovo* vaccination, i.e. vaccinating the embryonating egg (active acquired immunity prior to hatching).

The eventual success of any vaccination programme depends entirely on the thought and planning given to its formulation. While many individuals simply ask 'What vaccine should I use, and when should I use it?', a successful outcome demands that several questions are asked—and answered—in this order:

1. Are certain diseases present on this farm, or in my company? Or are my birds significantly at risk of contracting these diseases? If so, are these diseases a problem that warrants my company's investment in a committed, coordinated team effort at solving it (vaccine, labour, etc.)?

- With the exception of Marek's disease, never vaccinate your birds just because everyone else is vaccinating theirs. Once you've determined what pathogens are present on certain farms, and within your company, you must know specifically what strains, 'variants', or 'mutants' are present. The use of sentinel bird programmes will answer the questions about pathogens. With your help, good diagnostic assistance laboratories will answer these questions for you. Don't waste time and money vaccinating against agents and diseases that are not present in your bird's environment.

2. If disease is present in the birds, could vaccination prevent this problem, and is vaccination, therefore, necessary? If the answer is yes, is a vaccine against the agent commercially available, or must an autogenous vaccine be developed?

- Again, diagnostic consultants will help you answer these specific questions.
3. When are the chick's maternal antibody levels low enough to ensure successful vaccination via the chick's ability to respond immunologically to the vaccine in a calculated manner?
- Administer a vaccine when you *know* it will work. Guesswork costs too much time, money, and effort.
4. Which product shall be used on the birds, and how shall it be administered to them?
- If you know the answer to questions 1, 2 and 3, you will automatically know the answer to this question.

The point of asking these questions is to gather data that will allow you to find correct answers, save time, money and bird lives, and maximize profits.

Vaccine failure

The term 'vaccine failure' is generally meant to convey the idea that a particular vaccine failed to protect members of a flock from a disease. Because every vaccine lot is tested for potency, it is highly doubtful that the vaccine itself is actually ever responsible for a lack of immune response. So-called 'failure' almost always can be traced to improper handling and use of the vaccine (Tables 5.6 and 5.7).

Table 5.6 Mechanism of vaccine failures associated with certain biological events

Biological event	Mechanism of failure
Maternal antibodies present	Antigen–antibody reaction causes interference
Birds under stress	Disease present in flock Overcrowded conditions Poor nutritional status
Genetic features	Birds are genetic 'low responders'

When live vaccines are used, a mild or subclinical infection is being induced in the flock. The purpose is to create a mild form of the disease with minimal adverse effects under controlled conditions. Vaccinations are stressful events, with adverse reactions ranging from decreased appetite to death.

Compared to injected vaccines, inhaled or imbibed vaccines contain less virus on a per-chick basis. Therefore, if vaccination technique is not impeccable, chicks vaccinated by the water or coarse spray methods are less likely to receive an adequate dose of vaccine. 'Undervaccinated' chicks acquire the

Table 5.7 Possible causes of vaccine 'failure' arising during shipping, storage and administration

Shipping	Poor temperature control
	Damaged packing
Storage	Poor ventilation
	Poor temperature control
	Contamination by microbes or chemicals
Administration	Mixing products
	Using too low a dose
	Using incorrect route

vaccine virus from vaccinated flockmates. Because bird-to-bird transmission of vaccine viruses increases pathogenicity, this produces an extended 'rolling' reaction as chicks become infected at different times with virus of increased pathogenicity. While this is taking place, levels of protective maternal antibodies are declining in the chicks, making them more susceptible to infection.

Vaccination guidelines

General guidelines for vaccination include:

1. Never vaccinate birds that show overt signs of illness.
2. Use the manufacturer's recommended dose. There is an antigenic threshold that must be achieved by administering a prescribed amount of antigen necesssary to trigger antibody production. If the necessary amount is not administered the chicken will not produce sufficient antibodies. For this reason, vaccines should not be diluted beyond the vaccine manufacturer's recommendations.
3. The vaccines should be stored and handled according to the manufacturer's recommendations. Usually this means they should be refrigerated at 2–5 °C (35–45 °F) until used. Live lyophilized ('freeze-dried') vaccines should be reconstituted using the manufacturer's recommendations immediately before vaccinating a flock. The reconstitution liquid (diluent) provided with the lyophilized product (vaccine) is sterile, but the vaccine organisms begin to inactivate within a short period of time following rehydration. Therefore, after vaccinating a flock of chickens, left-over vaccines of this type should never be saved for later use, even under refrigeration, because the vaccine agents have been inactivated and are no longer capable of stimulating immunity in the chickens.

A common error is to reconstitute a lyophilized vaccine using chlorinated tap water. Not only is tap water not sterile, but the chlorine immediately kills the vaccine agent. Thus the vaccination is ineffective.

Vaccination methods

Methods of vaccination are simple, yet each step is important. The basic steps for common methods are outlined below.

Water vaccination—use of a medication tank

A simple sequence of events must take place when vaccines are administered via medication tanks into water troughs, bell drinkers, nipples or cups:

1. Remove drinking water 1 hour (hot weather) or 2–3 hours (normal conditions) before the vaccination to 'water-starve' the chicks.
2. Wash and scrub waterer to get rid of all soil and foreign matter. *Do not* use a sanitizing agent or disinfectant. Rinse well with clean water.
3. Use only clean pure water for the administration of vaccines. The quality of this water should have been determined previously. Never use chlorinated water for vaccination.
4. Use the vaccine properly according to the manufacturer's written instructions.
5. Prepare a mixture of 33 g dry skim milk in 1 litre (2 pints) of water. Add this preparation to 20 litres (5 gal) of water. The dry skim milk will neutralize any chemical residues that might inactivate the virus, and protects the vaccine from deterioration or inactivation.
6. Mix vaccine and skimmed milk/water mixture in a clean large bucket. Administer to the flock by pouring the mixture into the previously cleaned water troughs.
7. Following reconstitution, administer the vaccine immediately in *all* water troughs or throughout the water lines. To ensure that all birds drink, the flock should be gently moved and circulated ('stirred') by having workers walk slowly up through birds along one side of the house and down along the other.
8. Vaccine water ideally should be consumed by the flock within 20 minutes. If not, wait for it to be consumed, then turn on the water.
9. Vaccination date, manufacturer's serial number and any other pertinent information should be written on the flock's permanent health record.

Water vaccination—use of a proportioning (metering) device

A proportioner is a device for releasing metered amounts of a concentrated solution into the drinking water. The use of some watering devices may necessitate the use of a proportioner. Unfortunately, proportioners may be inconsistent in delivery and metering may be too high, too low, or not at all, and we do not recommend this method. Proportioners should be tested periodically to ensure that the proper, constant delivery of vaccine mixture is maintained. As with other equipment the proportioner manufacturer's recommendations should be followed. The main principles discussed in the previous section also apply in this section as well.

Spray vaccination

Spray vaccinators are employed at hatcheries and on farms to immunize chicks. This is done by spraying chicks individually (ocular or oral spray, or both), or by placing large groups of chicks in a flow-through spray cabinet, or by spraying the vaccine mixture on chicks as the vaccinator walks through the house. For each technique, the proper droplet size and volume must be delivered to the individual chick otherwise vaccination and immunization will not take place. The basic principles of immunization alluded to previously also apply to spray vaccination. Generally, a coarse spray ($< 50 \, \mu m$) is recommended for initial (priming) vaccination of young chicks or for vaccines with greater virulence (e.g. infectious laryngotracheitis virus, LaSota Newcastle, or low-passage infectious bronchitis virus). Fine sprays usually are reserved for use in older chicks, or for subsequent (booster) vaccination. Spray machinery must be periodically calibrated to ensure that droplet size is uniform and of the correct size. As for all other machines, service and maintenance schedules must be followed.

Portable backpack type sprayers have also been used to administer vaccines to older birds. A major pitfall to this method is poor distribution of the vaccine-laden aerosol, and birds either are not vaccinated or are overdosed and experience adverse reactions. Droplet size can be hard to regulate, and periodic checks must be made to ensure that proper droplet size and uniformity is being produced. In poultry houses, remember to turn off ventilation fans for a prescribed period of time when vaccines are being applied by spray. In open-sided houses, curtains must be up during spraying and for 45 minutes after spraying. On warm days, vaccination should be done during the cool morning hours. While one person slowly walks up the centre of the house to separate the chicks, two people with sprayers should follow, one on each side of and slightly behind the centre person.

Eyedrop vaccination

The general principles of vaccine and diluent handling and storage apply here too. When this method is used, every bird must be vaccinated, and each bird must be handled with care to prevent trauma. Damage to the cornea must be avoided. A mist or drop of vaccine is sprayed onto or allowed to fall onto the surface of the eyeball. The vaccinator tip must *never* touch the bird.

Parenteral vaccination

This vaccination technique is performed on individual chicks in the hatchery by workers who are trained to operate the special equipment. The main disadvantage is the time required to perform the individual injections, which makes it quite labour intensive. The principles of cleanliness and the delivery of the proper amount of vaccine as described previously apply. Vaccination equipment should be periodically calibrated and serviced in order to ensure that suitable mechanical delivery of vaccine into the chicks is taking place.

Vaccination crews

Vaccination crews are employed because they are efficient. A major problem is that without biosecurity they may cause more diseases than they prevent. The principles of biosecurity described above must therefore apply.

Vaccination analysis programme

Vaccination of flocks of birds entails evaluation of the success or failure of the vaccine programme. Firstly, vaccine quality and accuracy in packaging must be controlled and monitored. The poultry producer should be assured that what has been paid for is actually present in the vial of vaccine. If poultry company quality assurance or health services laboratories are not equipped and staffed to accomplish this task, institutional and private laboratories usually will have the resources to provide this service.

Secondly, breeder management must produce a healthy chick free of disease and in a physical condition that will enable it to respond to vaccination. By ascertaining the antibody levels following vaccination, the producer can deduce whether the programme is successful, if necessary by employing institutional or private laboratories. Another concern is whether the level of antibody is sufficient to prevent infection. Surprisingly, there are no industry-wide standard recommendations of protective antibody level. Therefore the empirical method of deciding if the level is adequate is based upon the performance of the chicks as they grow to market age.

Determination of performance includes, for example, achievement of predicted weight gain, feed conversion, mortality rate or absence or presence of other diseases. This may be complicated by environmental conditions and other management factors that influence chick health. For example, poor ventilation and ammonia build-up will result in respiratory diseases. If virus isolation demonstrates that Newcastle disease virus is present, the wrong conclusion of 'vaccine failure' may be made. The isolated virus might only have been the vaccine virus itself!

Evaluating immunity

There are many serological tests—enzyme-linked immunosorbent assay (ELISA), virus neutralization (VN), hemagglutination inhibition (HI), etc.— that are available to estimate the individual chicken's degree of immunity (antibody level). The basic problem is how many samples are necessary to provide a true antibody picture of the flock and what these results mean in practical terms. To give results that one can interpret with confidence, *at least* 15 serum samples from any group of chicks should be tested.

Recognizing that the efficacy of vaccines will probably not be determined by the direct challenge method, another method of analysis has been successfully developed. Called Vaccine Analysis Program (VAP) by its originators, the basis for VAP is quite simple. Customized for each company, the protective antibody levels (titres) to the various vaccines are monitored and used to define normal levels of protection. New samples are monitored on a schedule and compared to the baseline to determine if the antibody levels of the sample are acceptable or not. This 'yes or no' answer eliminates guesswork and confusion and immediately informs the health manager if his vaccination programme is working and how well it is working. Computerized for quick comparisons, a graph shows whether antibody titres are acceptable or not. Poultry companies who do not use this or a similar analysis programme are wasting time and money.

Medication: types and usage

As with vaccinations, medication of sick birds is no substitute for good disease prevention programmes. In fact, when medication of birds becomes a necessity, the producer has already incurred the following:

1. Reduced body weight gain
2. Suboptimal pigmentation or colour

3. Labour and drug costs
4. Morbidity and mortality
5. Condemnations and/or lower grades (downgrades) of carcases at inspection.

Medications are formulated to be delivered in the feed or the water, although water medication is preferred because often sick birds will not eat but will continue to drink. Specific drugs, antibiotics, or anthelmintics used in the treatment of diseases will not be discussed here as recommended therapies change often, or may not be appropriate under all conditions. Additionally, dosage and withdrawal times, which are usually specified on the manufacturer's label, differ depending upon country of origin or use. In the USA and other countries, government inspection agencies constantly conduct assays of slaughtered poultry for illegal tissue levels of drugs, antibiotics and other chemical residues. Common causes of illegal residues include:

1. Failure to follow instructions concerning withdrawal times
2. Feed mill mistakes
3. Feed delivery mistakes
4. Intentional misuse of medications.

However, proper administration of drugs and parasiticides when required is essential to minimize disease and condemnations. Central to the issue is public concern over drug and pesticide usage and any persistent levels that might remain in the carcase. Therefore it is both necessary and prudent for the industry to use drugs sparingly and appropriately.

When chickens are sick, veterinarians must diagnose the disease quickly and correctly and respond with the appropriate treatment, at the recommended level, for the recommended period of time. Inadequate dosages or improper medication can:

1. Allow the course of the disease to continue unabated
2. Allow the disease to spread
3. Confuse the character of the disease leading to a wrong diagnosis, or to peculiar or enhanced signs, or
4. Require the further application and expenditure of medicaments, procedures and labour.

When birds are sick they eat less. One unfortunate scenario is of lower consumption of feed containing a coccidiostat leading to an outbreak of coccidiosis in addition to the primary disease. Conversely, an increase in medicated food or water consumption (such as increased water consumption during hot weather) can result in drug toxicity.

Since medications are either delivered in the feed or in the water it is wise to retain samples of each delivery of feed. These samples should be placed in clean *paper* (not plastic, glass, or foil) bags which should have the date of delivery. These should be refrigerated and kept until the birds have been processed.

Water quantity and quality

Chicks that have ample clean air, water and food will grow at a profitable rate. Water is the single most important nutrient for poultry. To illustrate this fact, chicks can lose 98% of their body fat or 50% of body protein and still survive. But a 10% loss in body water will result in serious physiological illness, and a 20% loss will result in death. Although intermittent watering or water restriction can be successful in some poultry settings (e.g. pullets and laying hens), such programmes have never been successful in broiler production.

The farm's water source should be analysed for colour, turbidity, hardness, iron, pH, solid materials, nitrogen, poisons and bacteria, at least annually. Always test water at its source. Acceptable limits for material in drinking water are listed in Table 5.8, and the chief criteria are considered below:

1. Colour. Any colour is due to certain substances in solution, such as tannins or tannic acid, iron salts, etc.
2. Turbidity. Particles such as silt or bacteria in suspension rather than in solution cause the water to be turbid.
3. Hardness. Salts of calcium (Ca) and magnesium (Mg) form scale and sludge and cause water to be 'hard' which affects the taste. Also, solubility of medications can be altered in excessively hard or soft water.

   Excessive water hardness may have an adverse effect on water-administered vaccines, medications, disinfectants, detergents and cleaners. Calcium carbonate deposits will build up on water system components and appliances. In extreme cases and over time, water flow rates will be reduced. The use of chemical compounds such as polyphosphates will increase the solubility of Ca and Mg and prevent the accumulation of gelatinous sludge or scaly materials that will clog watering systems.

   Conversely, water softness may be a problem when magnesium or sodium is greater than 50 parts per million (ppm), especially when chlorine is greater than 14 ppm.
4. Iron. Although iron in water seldom affects chickens, at high concentrations it imparts a bitter taste and it stains almost everything with

Table 5.8 Acceptable limits for drinking water criteria in poultry

Property or material	Upper limit	Comments
Bacteria	0 cfu[1]/ml	Presence of some bacteria may not cause problems. Coliforms indicate faecal contamination
Nitrates[2]	20 ppm[3]	At 3–20 ppm adverse effects occur. Above 20 ppm performance declines
Phosphorus (P)	–[4]	Upper limit for poultry not established. For humans upper limit is 0.1 ppm
Potassium (K)	–	Upper limit for poultry not established
Calcium (Ca)	600 ppm	May improve feed conversion and body weight gain, but decreases liveability
Magnesium (Mg)	125 ppm	At this level, has laxative effects
Manganese (Mn)	0.05 ppm	May form black deposits on equipment, promotes leaking in components such as valves
Iron (Fe)	25 ppm	Water has metallic taste, stains equipment
Aluminium (Al)	–	Upper limit for poultry not established. For humans upper limit is 0.05 ppm
Zinc (Zn)	5.0 ppm	Water has bitter taste
Sodium (Na)	50 ppm	Causes diarrhoea (loose droppings)
Hardness	110 ppm	Interferes with many disinfectants, biologicals and medications

[1] cfu = colony forming unit.
[2] It is not unusual in the UK for borehole water sources to exceed 50 ppm.
[3] ppm = parts per million.
[4] Toxic limit not known.

which it comes in contact. Problems with high iron and manganese levels can be effectively reduced or eliminated by using chlorinators, filters or water softeners.

5. pH. The pH of a solution is a measure of its acidity or alkalinity. When above 7, it is alkaline; below 7, it is acid. Water normally has a pH of about 7–7.2. A pH of 8.0 (10 times more alkaline than pH 7.0) is considered to be the upper limit for poultry. A pH of 6.4 is considered to be the lower limit.

Reduced production performance is encountered when pH drops below 6.4. Low pH can cause corrosion of metal parts in watering systems, and may also compound other water quality problems, making it more difficult to remove high levels of minerals. The pH of excessively acidic water can be raised by utilizing neutralizing filters or installing a soda ash injecting system. If filters are used, they should be checked at least weekly and replaced when necessary. High pH can be corrected by adding a proper level of food grade phosphoric acid to the water.

6. Total solid materials. Total solids represent the total amount of solid material in a suspension or solution.

7. Nitrates, nitrites. High nitrate and nitrite levels indicate that decaying organic material is present, therefore levels are used as an indirect indicator of contamination. Nitrates are not easily removed from a water supply. Distillation, reverse osmosis and ion-exchange can be used to eliminate nitrates but they are very expensive. It is easier, and cheaper, to keep nitrate contamination out of the water supply than to remove it once it is there.

8. Toxic metal compounds (e.g. lead, cadmium, copper, arsenic, mercury, aluminium). When present in excess of 0.5 ppm, many of these elements may accumulate in the bird and illness often results.

9. Bacteria. The presence of certain genera of bacteria in drinking water is undesirable, and generally indicates that faecal contamination of the water source is taking place. The type of bacteria, rather than number, is important in water analysis. Some bacteria may be detrimental to human beings and chickens. This is particularly true for the coliform bacteria, such as *Escherichia coli*.

Enclosed watering systems increase water quality by reducing bacterial contamination. Shallow wells, lakes, rivers, streams and ponds are usually not good sources of high quality water without some form of water treatment. This is because bacteria and nitrates are picked up from surrounding pastures by surface water. Wells should be deep, and must be capped with at least a 60 cm (2 ft) diameter concrete slab. This will stop surface water from running down the casing and into the well.

Bacterial contamination can be eliminated by removing the source of contamination, or by filtration and/or chlorination. Wells can be 'shock' chlorinated by adding 56 g (2 oz) 50% chlorine solution for every 113 l (25 gal) of water in the well. Commercial bleach is 5.25% chlorine (sodium hypochlorite), so 540 g (19 oz) of bleach will equal 56 g of 50% chlorine. After 2–3 hours to allow the chlorine to disperse in the well water, chlorinated water should be pumped into the water system and allowed to stand for 6–8 hours to disinfect pipes, equipment, etc. Flush the system completely to remove all chlorine odour before housing chicks. An inexpensive swimming pool chlorine test kit can be used to determine how much residual chlorine is in the drinking water.

Chlorinating devices periodically inject a metered amount of chlorine into the circulating water system. Continuous chlorination at 1–3 ppm will reduce numbers of microorganisms, litter moisture and litter caking, but it may not significantly increase broiler performance. However, higher levels of chlorine can decrease water consumption and decrease body weight gain.

Live vaccines and bacteria are killed by chlorine and chlorinated water, so chlorination of water should be discontinued at least 3 days before and for 3 days after administering any live biological products. If the drinking water supply is municipal water (and, therefore, is chlorinated water), then vaccine should be mixed in a solution of 85–113 g (3–4 oz) dried non-fat milk in 22.5 l (5 gal) of water. Milk will help protect the vaccine by neutralizing the chlorine.

Enclosed watering systems reduce, but do not eliminate, the chore of cleaning out the system. In fact, systems that incorporate nipple-type drinkers demand that managers spend time and effort knowing how the system operates, and making sure that the system operates properly. Failure to do so means that optimal broiler performance can be crippled. For example, in enclosed water systems, pressure must be regulated and periodically monitored. Excessive high or low pressure will result in birds who either cannot get enough water or get excessive water and damp litter under the drinkers.

Differential diagnosis of respiratory disease

Physiological overview

Elsewhere in this chapter we have emphasized the deleterious effects of ammonia and other gases on poultry. This is due to the size, structure, form and function of the avian respiratory system.

Firstly, when compared to mammalian lungs, the lungs of the chicken are proportionally smaller. Secondly, the avian lung utilizes capillaries for the flow of air as well as blood. This makes the avian lung more efficient but also makes the bird more sensitive to toxic gases than mammals. A well-known example of this is the practice of 19th-century miners who took canaries into the mines as biological poisonous gas detectors. Similarly, Allied military forces in Europe and the Persian Gulf took chickens into the theatre of operations where chemical weapons might be used against humans.

Avian white blood cells are less efficient at ingesting debris and killing infectious agents than their mammalian counterparts. These agents can thus accumulate quickly to reach dangerous levels in the avian respiratory system.

It is not possible to diagnose respiratory disease by simple physical examination. Regardless of the cause, birds commonly exhibit a range of respiratory signs, like sneezing, breathing hard, snicking, coughing, etc.

In order to prevent and control disease, one must have excellent diagnostic facilities and techniques (Figure 5.1). An accurate diagnosis requires a good medical history and appropriate laboratory test results. Old adages such as 'A history well taken is a diagnosis half made' and 'Mysterious illness usually is

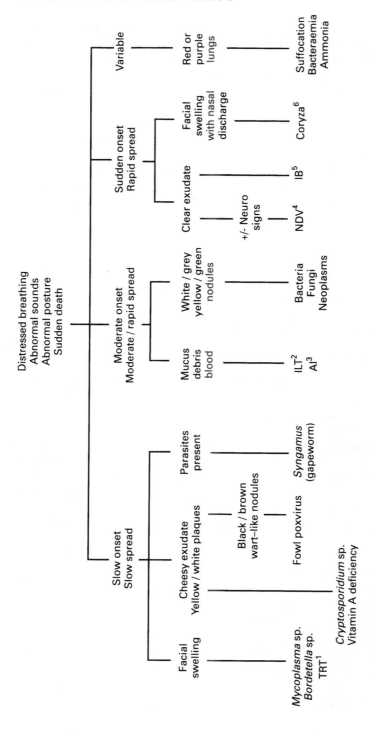

Figure 5.1 An algorithm for diagnosis of common respiratory diseases of broilers.

1 Turkey rhinotracheitis
2 Infectious laryngotracheitis (herpesvirus)
3 Avian influenza (orthomyxovirus)
4 Newcastle disease virus (paramyxovirus)
5 Infectious bronchitis (coronavirus)
6 *Haemophilus gallinarum*

the result of inadequate diagnostics' are predominantly true. This illustrates the need for keeping proper records.

Good record forms which can be customized for a particular operation are widely available. Modern record keeping also involves retrieval of management and disease information via computer. Computerized information allows comparisons to be made with flexibility and speed that would be impractical with ordinary manual record systems, making it possible to determine objectively the results of managerial decisions. For example, the association between poor litter conditions, disease conditions and diminished profitability can be related and graphically illustraated. This also is the purpose of Vaccine Analysis Program, alluded to previously, which is used to determine the efficiency of a vaccination programme.

Many diagnoses are missed or incorrectly made because the proper samples were not obtained and diagnostic procedures were not consistently performed. There is a great chasm between a presumptive and a confirmed diagnosis. Specifically for a case of respiratory disease the following should be performed:

1. A complete medical history should be taken.
2. Paired blood (serum) samples should be collected for serological testing.
3. Cultures (bacterial, viral, chlamydial and mycoplasmal) from organs with gross lesions should be collected aseptically.
4. Cytologies (touch imprint or scraping) should be taken from affected organs to determine the presence/absence of agents such as *Cryptosporidium*.
5. Histopathology, including ultrastructure from organs with lesions, should be requested.

This information, properly integrated, permits an informed and, therefore, intelligent diagnosis.

It is too simplistic to ascribe a disease to a causative agent. Viruses such as NDV, IBV and IBD are uniquitously present in the environment, yet not all flocks or all individuals in a flock become diseased. The reason for this is clear: while the disease agent must be present, for disease to occur other environmental factors must be present or absent. Obviously, ventilation is a key factor (see Chapter 2). Not only should it provide adequate oxygen, but it should also dilute airborne disease organisms and remove harmful gases and excessive moisture. Prevention of respiratory disease requires an environment where damage to the respiratory tract does not occur. A healthy bird in a properly ventilated environment will resist the pathogenic organisms normally present in the environment.

Ventilation

Proper ventilation of poultry houses is a major requirement for producing healthy chickens. During the warmer months ventilation aids in reducing environmental temperature. It also reduces excess humidity and prevents moisture build-up. However, in efforts to maintain high poultry house temperatures while conserving energy costs and keeping production costs low, producers often restrict ventilation. This is a false economy because proper ventilation provides fresh moving air to both supply oxygen to the bird and to help remove the build-up of harmful gases such as carbon dioxide and ammonia.

Ammonia is produced in damp excreta-rich litter. It is a harmful gas because it damages the eyes and respiratory organs (sinuses, trachea, lungs and air sacs). This damage reduces ciliary action in the trachea, diminishing the rate of clearance of mucus, bacteria, viruses and dust from the tract. As a result, the chicken's ability to defend itself against pathogens such as Newcastle disease virus and *Escherichia coli* (Plate 3) is reduced. Pneumonia and airsacculitis commonly result from high ammonia levels (e.g. 20 ppm) in poorly ventilated poultry houses. Very high concentrations of ammonia in the air (40 ppm) can actually cause blindness. Reliable and accurate ammonia sensors have been developed. These instruments should be used routinely as part of an overall air quality assurance programme.

Ventilation systems

It is beyond the scope of this chapter to prescribe the details of proper ventilation programmes for broilers. Engineers who understand poultry farming needs have designed poultry houses which are properly ventilated for the climatic extremes of the geographic area in mind. They should be consulted for their electrical, physical and mechanical expertise.

We cannot overemphasize the basic importance of ventilation and how poor control results in respiratory disease. A correctly ventilated environment for poultry can be costly, yet still be cost effective. The question is cost effectiveness. During the winter a tightly enclosed house that traps gases, moisture and pathogens costs more in terms of disease than expenses saved by lowered energy costs. Here are some general considerations for effective ventilation:

1. The system should be designed to provide proper ventilation during climatic extremes.
2. The manufacturer's recommendations and specifications should be followed.
3. Overcrowding of birds should be avoided to prevent exceeding the ventilation capacity.

4. Ventilation equipment should be cleaned and maintained on a regular schedule both to provide optimal effectiveness and to extend the life of the system. This should be done minimally between grow-outs but ideally about every 30 days, and whenever accumulation dust and dirt become visible. The ventilation system should be checked in order to determine if it is performing at the level designed.

5. A reliable alarm system in the event of a power failure and an automatic start-up generator should be used.

Selected important diseases of broilers

Escherichia coli infection

Large numbers of *E. coli* organisms are produced in the intestines of poultry. There may be as many as one million organisms/gram of faeces. There are many different strains of the organism and they can be classified by their O, H and K antigens. The majority are non-pathogenic, but a small proportion, especially types O_1, O_2 and O_{78} can produce disease in poultry.

Disease caused by *E. coli* infection is probably the most common and economically significant problem in broilers world-wide. This is not only in terms of mortality, but also in the effects of loss of growth, poor feed conversion and downgrading after processing.

As a normal inhabitant of the intestinal tract, the numbers of *E. coli* organisms in the environment of the poultry house can build up very rapidly. The organisms can survive better in dry conditions and are harboured in large numbers in litter and dust.

Route of infection

There are two routes of infection which produce different disease conditions. Firstly, the presence of *E. coli* in faeces can result in the contamination of the shell of hatching eggs, resulting in yolk sac infection as described in Chapter 3. Secondly, *E. coli* also infects poultry by the respiratory route. This usually occurs in broilers between 4 and 6 weeks of age, as a result of dust buildup and the birds' rapidly increasing requirements for air.

Lesions

Respiratory infection results in haemorrhagic tracheitis and pneumonia, with air sacculitis involving the abdominal and thoracic air sacs. Associated inflammation of the pericardium and the surface of the liver occurs. The air sacs and pericardium appear thickened and cloudy and there is usually a fibrinous membrane covering the surface of the liver. The spleen is enlarged, dark and congested. Birds generally die in good bodily condition and there is often an extensive discolouration of the muscles over the pectoral region, giving a light/dark patchy appearance. The septicaemia can sometimes produce other lesions, for example joint infections, dermatitis and osteomyelitis.

Predisposing factors

There are many important factors which predispose to respiratory infection with *E. coli*.

1. Ammonia buildup in the poultry house can be extremely harmful. Levels above 20 ppm affect growth performance, but also the gas has a direct effect on the respiratory tract. It interferes with the action of the cilia lining the trachea and increases mucus production. This means that the mucus stream is not cleared properly from the respiratory tract and acts as a site for bacterial multiplication. Ammonia also decreases the activity of macrophages which are phagocytic cells available for engulphing bacteria in the submucosa of the trachea. Rotating litter may not be a good idea if it results in the release of large quantities of trapped ammonia from beneath the surface of the litter.
2. Dust may contain 20 000–800 000 *E. coli* organisms/gram. Dust buildup makes it more likely for *E. coli* infection to occur. Adequate ventilation is vital to ensure removal and dilution of both dust and ammonia. Proper and flexible control of ventilation is probably the most significant factor in control of respiratory disease.
3. With large quantities of dust in houses, drinking water can become contaminated particularly if the header tank is not covered. If high levels of *E. coli* build up in drinking water supplies, it is generally detrimental to bird health.
4. A poor standard of farm hygiene will allow the buildup of *E. coli* in the environment. The clean out after each crop should be extremely thorough, including not only floors, walls and ceilings, but also fan shafts, ventilation ducts and the surrounds of the house. A thorough disinfection should also include the header tank and drinking water system.
5. *E. coli* infection often follows infection with a virus affecting the respiratory system or the use of live vaccine. Newcastle disease and infectious bronchitis are particularly important in this respect. *Mycoplasma gallisep-*

ticum and *M. synoviae* are also important predisposing causes of *E. coli* infection.

6. Any form of stress will exacerbate *E. coli* infection, for example over-stocking, or extremes of heat and cold have an adverse effect.

7. The size of the poultry unit, the number of houses on the site and the relation of the site to other poultry farms are important factors in determining the buildup of *E. coli* infection.

Prevention

As has been mentioned before, the respiratory disease is often a complex of *E. coli* which interacts with virus or *Mycoplasma* infection and can be exacerbated by various environmental factors. When a diagnosis of coli septicaemia has been made it is tempting to start the flock on a course of antibiotic treatment immediately. However, it is most important to study the factors which precipitated the outbreak in the first place. In controlled environment housing a study of air movement and ventilation control will pay dividends. Sometimes air exchange will seem adequate and the air comfortable to breathe at human height, but bending down to bird level will reveal a stale and torpid atmosphere. It is *vital* that air is circulating freely just above the litter where the birds are situated. As well as assisting breathing and reducing the numbers of bacteria, the air helps to remove excess moisture from the litter which favours buildup of *E. coli* infection.

Treatment

When the lesions of septicaemia including pericarditis and perihepatitis are seen, a presumptive diagnosis of coli septicaemia can be made. Cultures should be made from liver and heart blood and plated out on blood agar and violet red bile agar on MacConkey, which is selective for *E. coli* organisms. It is essential to rule out organisms such as *Salmonella* and *Pasteurella* which can also cause septicaemia. To save time, a sensitivity test may be carried out on the primary culture. The antibiotics included on the discs should be chlortetracycline, oxytetracycline, trimethoprim, sulphaquinoxaline, furazolidone, amoxycillin and lincospectin. Neomycin is not much use for treating septicaemia because of its poor gut absorption. Other drugs if available such as the quinolones (flumequin) may also be tested. The sensitivity test result should be available the next day and treatment should be initiated using the most cost effective antibiotic. For example, if the culture shows sensitivity to furazolidone and lincospectin, it would be sensible to use the cheaper furazolidone. For acute infections it is usual to treat in the drinking water first as sick birds will generally drink even though they may not be eating. This is followed, after say three days, with treatment in feed for a further period of 3–5 days depending on the circumstances. Obviously if birds are near to slaughter and there is a five day withdrawal on a drug, it is necessary to stop treatment to ensure there are no tissue residues in the meat.

For water treatment a proportioner is the best way of adding the medication to the water. Usually one is not available, so it is essential to know the birds' daily water consumption and the volume of the header tank. The antibiotic should be thoroughly dissolved in a small quantity of water first before adding to the header tank. Always watch for blockages in pipes or drinkers that may be caused by dirt or algae dislodged by the addition of the antibiotic to the water. Try and medicate three or four times during the day.

In feed treatment is generally easier and more reliable, but to be immediately effective the feed bin must obviously be empty. Here it helps to have two bins for each house. This method is especially useful if a course of preventive medication is being used, for example in anticipation of an outbreak of coli septicaemia based on previous flock history.

It must be remembered that treatment is generally ineffective for yolk sac infection, and tends to prolong the condition rather than cure it. Thus it is not recommended.

Continued use of one antibiotic on one farm should be discouraged. Instead a change of antibiotic is advised. It is to be hoped that treatment would not be needed on a regular basis on any one farm, as it is usually a sign of some fundamental weakness such as poor ventilation, bad hygiene or poor vaccination practice.

In some organizations, routine medication is included in chick starter to try and overcome any egg-borne *E. coli* infection and to help the early growth of the chick. However, to recommend such a programme is an admission of failure, as chicks should be of good enough quality not to need antibiotic in the starter. Also the use of antibiotic in this way could make that antibiotic unavailable for treatment when it may be more urgently required later in the life of the flock.

Factory condemnations

Sometimes the first indication of a buildup of *E. coli* infection on a farm may be an increase in the number condemned for septicaemia at processing. This number should not normally be higher than 0.5% and certainly above 1% indicates there is a problem. It is surprising that numbers as great as this can occur sometimes without there being clinical signs of respiratory disease on the farm.

Other conditions associated with E. coli

- In broilers a complication of infectious bronchitis or other virus respiratory disease may lead to facial oedema with sinusitis, from which *E. coli* can be isolated as a secondary infection. Swollen head syndrome was first described in South Africa, but is now commonly seen in the UK and some other countries.
- A condition in broiler breeders has also been given the name swollen head syndrome. In this case, along with the facial swelling there is usually discharge from the ear and marked nervous signs including opisthotonus. *E. coli* can be isolated from the brains and lesions of egg peritonitis which are generally present. These birds have recently been found to convert serologically positive to the turkey rhinotracheitis virus.
- Egg peritonitis, with *E. coli* infection, is the most common cause of mortality in laying birds around the period of maximum egg laying.

Conclusion

E. coli infections are very common in poultry and take many forms. Their control can be as much a test of management skill as veterinary diagnosis and preventive medicine.

Leg weakness/lameness of broiler chickens

The following is a descriptive list of the commonest causes of leg weakness in broilers. Very little systematic study has been carried out to identify the level of incidence of the various conditions and the figures quoted below are based on small commercial or research studies. The conditions are presented in three groups indicating, in descending order, their relative importance within the industry.

Group 1

Angular bone deformity

A complex deformity of the lower leg, due to combinations of rotation of the distal tibio-tarsus with or without either lateral (valgus) or medial (varus)

169

bending of the bones above and below the hock. The cause is complex with genetics, exercise, environment, food quantity and composition all appearing to have an influence. A reduction in the incidence has been demonstrated by restricting food intake and altering standard light patterns both of which are likely to induce more activity. Incidence is normally in the range of 0.5–2% but may reach 5–25% in problem flocks.

Tibial dyschondroplasia

This condition is characterized by the persistence of an abnormal mass of cartilage in the metaphysis below the growth plate of long bones. It occurs most commonly in the proximal end of the tibio-tarsus in which site the severest lesions are seen, but also appears in the metatarsus in approximately one-third of cases. Lameness is usually seen only in those affected birds which develop bowing due to necrosis or fractures of the long bones adjacent to the abnormal cartilage. Incidence can be 30% or more but most of these birds are affected subclinically. A strong genetic influence has been demonstrated associated with selection for early and rapid growth, although the aetiology is also influenced by management factors, in particular, nutrition. Severe food restriction will reduce the incidence but the degree of restriction needed to achieve satisfactory results may make this impractical as a method of control. Recent research has shown that addition of a vitamin D metabolite can reduce the incidence or severity of the lesions.

Femoral head necrosis

There appear to be several causes leading to this condition, which is a general term describing a variety of gross lesions in the femoral head and proximal femur. These lesions may be seen in batches of birds from the same house and losses of up to 3% may be experienced. Affected birds exhibit an unsteady gait which develops to severe lameness. In one form the femoral head disintegrates completely, becomes brown and discoloured and the neck of the femur is brittle. This form is seen at about 4–5 weeks of age.

Another form involves an infarction in the femoral head caused by vascular occlusion of the growth plate cartilage leading to epiphyseolysis. Detachment of the proximal femoral cartilaginous epiphyis has also been reported both in the growing bird and at slaughter. It is thought that this occurs because of repeated trauma and strictly should not be considered as femoral head necrosis unless there is concurrent degeneration of the protruding proximal end of the femur.

Suggested causes are bacterial infection (osteomyelitis), osteoporosis and malabsorption (runting and stunting) syndrome. Incidence may be related to the older types of housing which are more difficult to effectively clean and disinfect between batches, suggesting an infectious cause for the condition. Antibiotic therapy for 5–7 days may be of value in the treatment of this condition.

Bacterial synovitis/arthritis/osteomyelitis

Synovitis. Inflammation of the tendon sheaths due to infection with usually *Staphylococcus aureus* or occasionally *Escherichia coli* and *Pseudomonas aeruginosa*. **Septic arthritis**. This is seen particularly in the hock joint and involving *S. aureus* or *Pasteurella multocida* infection. **Osteomyelitis**. Occasionally infection involving *Salmonella*, *E. coli* or *Staphylococcus* spreads to bone and bone marrow leading to an osteomyelitis which can produce severe lameness. These infectious disorders may sometimes be responsive to antibiotic therapy usually given for 5–7 days.

Hockburn/plantar pododermatitis

Erosions involving ulceration and necrosis of the skin of the hock/plantar surface of the foot. Evidence suggests that lesions are caused by a combination of contact dermatitis and pressure necrosis. It has been observed under three main conditions of the poultry litter surface, these being wet litter, greasy litter or high litter nitrogen. It can be alleviated by good management practices, including maintenance of friable litter by environmental control, and attention to nutrition such that excretion of excess water and poorly digested fats is minimized. Increasing the stocking density increases the risk of incidence as will the occurrence of debilitating disease. Recent work has shown that pododermatitis may be reduced by giving biotin supplement in the diet.

Group 2

Tenosynovitis (viral arthritis)

Inflammation of the flexor tendon sheath running along the tarsometatarsal, the sheaths of the gastrocnemius tendon above the point of the hock and often the hock joint itself. The causal agent is a reovirus. Rupture of the gastrocnemius, the so-called 'green leg' may occur as a sequel especially if the birds are taken to higher weights.

Perosis (so-called slipped tendon)

An enlargement and deformity of the bones of the tibio-metatarsal joint, with twisting or bending of the distal tibia and proximal tarsus, and finally slipping of the gastrocnemius tendon. Manganese (or choline) deficiency has been shown to be a possible cause. In some birds the gastrocnemius tendon can sometimes slip from its normal position leading to loss of control of the lower leg. This is not related to manganese or other deficiency.

Crooked toes

Twisting of the digits in either the medial or lateral direction. The incidence in a flock can be very high (50% or more) without much associated lameness. This should be differentiated from a condition where the toes curl ventrally due to degeneration of peripheral nerves. This latter condition has been shown to be caused by riboflavin deficiency and also a weakness of the hocks.

Spondylolisthesis (kinky back)

A deviation of the spinal column in the region of the sixth thoracic vertebra which leads to excessive pressure on the seventh vertebra. Up to 20% of a flock may show a degree of deformity without clinical signs. In severe cases spinal cord compression occurs resulting in bilateral leg weakness or paraplegia. The condition is not congenital but has an hereditary disposition occurring only in broilers which have a very high early growth rate. It occurs between 1–9 weeks of age with peak incidence at 3–6 weeks. Clinical incidence can be completely prevented by severe food restriction during the first two weeks of life.

Group 3

Scoliosis

A lateral deviation of the vertebral column, usually in the mid-thoracic region. This condition has a low incidence and rarely interferes with locomotion.

Infectious synovitis

An inflammation of all synovial membranes caused by *Mycoplasma synoviae*, also known as infectious arthritis, tendovaginitis and enlarged hock. The UK is thought to be clear of this condition.

Osteomalacia (rickets)

This condition is caused by a deficiency of vitamin D, phosphorus, or more rarely calcium. Seen as skeletal deformities particularly in the leg bones.

Infectious bursal disease (Gumboro disease)

This is described in Chapter 6 and is probably the most economically significant infectious disease of broilers in Europe. One, two or even three doses of vaccines are required for its control. Dosage regimes are very variable according to the area and the degree of challenge that may be experienced, so it is impossible to generalize on the best vaccination programme.

Marek's disease

This disease is also described in Chapter 6 and may be important in broilers where they are being kept to heavier weights greater than 60 days of age and also in countries such as the USA, which do not always clean out the houses after every crop of broilers.

Ascites

This condition is characterized by an accumulation of proteinaceous fluid in the abdominal cavity caused by failure of the right side of the heart. It used to be a condition seen mainly at high altitude as a result of increased pulmonary arterial pressure due to lower oxygen tension at high altitude. However, it is common now to see it at low altitude. Some believe that ascites may be a consequence of lowered oxygen tension in poultry sheds caused by increased quantities of dust or noxious fumes as a result of poor ventilation. It is known that the disease can be controlled by improving ventilation and slowing the growth of birds.

Sudden death syndrome (flip over disease, heart attacks)

This is a very common disease in young male broilers occurring principally between 3 and 6 weeks of age. Birds are found dead, lying on their back and it is quite normal for this to be the commonest cause of mortality in well-managed flocks where no other disease occurs.

Infectious stunting syndrome

This illness is characterized by failure to thrive, slow growth and feathering during the first few weeks of life. This is an infectious disease caused, at least in part, by several viruses. Musculoskeletal disease is a common sequella. The disease is more commonly seen in progeny from parent flocks in the first two months of lay. Lateral spread may occur, especially in conditions of poor hygiene and overstocking on broiler farms. Depending on the severity of the disease, birds may remain permanently stunted or may start to grow again but generally do not reach the expected weight for their age.

Necrotic enteritis

This disease occurs sporadically, but mortality can be very high in untreated flocks. Illness caused by the proliferation of *Clostridium perfringens* (type c) often occurs in association with outbreaks of coccidiosis or any other situation which causes damage to the lining of the intestine. For example it is known that certain types of fish meal containing high levels of biogenic amines can precipitate necrotic enteritis. The disease responds well to penicillin treatment either in the water or in the feed.

Gangrenous dermatitis

This disease also may be related to clostridial infection although *Staphylococcus aureus* has also been involved. There is a correlation with infectious bursal disease and the chicken anaemia virus.

Chicken anaemia virus

This disease, mentioned in Chapter 6, is caused by a virus which is egg transmitted usually from young parent flocks. Infection is sometimes manifest by a condition called blue wing disease where haemorrhage and necrosis are found on the wings and other parts of the body. This disease should not be confused with gangrenous dermatitis and generally occurs in birds up to 20 days old.

Respiratory disease

The differential diagnosis of common respiratory diseases is shown in Figure 5.1.

Further reading

Calnek B W (ed) (1991) *Diseases of poultry* 9th edn. Iowa State University Press (USA), Wolfe Publishing (outside USA), London.

Jordan F T W (ed) (1990) *Poultry diseases* 3rd edn. Baillière Tindall, London.

Farm Animal Welfare Council (1992) *Report on the Welfare of Broiler Chickens*. Ministry of Agriculture, Fisheries and Food, Surbiton, Surrey.

CHAPTER

DISEASE PREVENTION AND CONTROL IN BROILER BREEDERS AND LAYERS

MARK PATTISON BVSc, MSc, PhD, MRCVS, DPMP

Introduction
Management of broiler breeders
Feed control
Transfer to laying house
Response to disease
Medication
Management of layers
Important diseases of breeders and layers
Monitoring and vaccination programmes
Investigating a drop in egg production
Further reading

Introduction

The development of the modern broiler became possible with the importation of heavy lines from the USA to the UK and some other European countries in the late 1950s. As explained in Chapter 1 hybrid breeding of layers and broilers started at this time. As genetic progress has improved liveweight gain and feed conversion in the broiler, so it has been necessary in the breeders to ensure that there has been selection for egg numbers in the female lines and that the male lines have remained fit and capable of natural mating. As the body frame has increased in size, it has become necessary to control the weight of both female and male breeders so they do not become too fat and are able to mate and lay eggs successfully. Thus diet and feed quantity has to be carefully controlled. In layers, genetic progress has been enormously successful and again it is important that layers, especially those larger strains that lay brown eggs, do not become too fat, so that their egg production can be optimized.

Management of broiler breeders

Delivery

Day-old breeder chicks are delivered in a vehicle with controlled temperature from the specialist primary breeding company. The temperature of the lorry will have been carefully controlled to around 25 °C (77 °F) and it is important that on arrival, the chicks are unloaded quickly and placed under the brooders as soon as possible, to avoid chilling.

The chick boxes are normally labelled with the codes showing the identity of the flock of origin and their approximate age. It is desirable to brood chicks from different flocks separately, but whether this is possible will depend upon the layout of pens and houses on the rearing farm and the number of flocks of origin. Males are reared separately from females, allowing 3–4 birds/m^2 (2.5–3.5 ft^2/bird). Pullets are reared at 4–7 birds/m^2 (1.5–2.5 ft^2/bird).

Brooding

The house must be thoroughly cleaned and disinfected, with a 10–15 cm (4–6 in) layer of clean wood shavings on the floor, for the new intake of chicks. In some countries wood shavings may not be available, so rice hulls, chopped straw or paper may be used for litter.

The brooders are switched on for 12–24 h before the arrival of the chicks to ensure the correct temperature has been achieved in both the house and under the brooders. Chicks are normally started at a house temperature of 24 °C (75 °F) with 32 °C (90 °F) under the brooders. The temperature is reduced gradually to 18 °C (64 °F) by 28 days. If whole house brooding is used, it is important not to exceed 31 °C (88 °F) otherwise chicks can become dehydrated.

It is normal practice to use supplementary feeders and drinkers to give extra feeding and drinking space in the first few days of life to encourage the chicks to eat and drink. It helps to use tepid water in chick drinkers rather than cold water straight from the tap.

Lighting

It is important in controlled-environment housing to have good light control for rearing the birds, with as little light leakage as possible. As little as 0.4 lx (0.04 foot-candles) during the dark period can interfere with the programme. Chicks start on 24 hours of light reducing to 8 hours by 2 weeks of age. This is then held constant to 19 weeks of age.

In the UK, controlled-environment housing is generally used, but open-sided or windowed housing can also be used in hotter climates, and depending on the local day length conditions and the time of the year, a specific programme is designed. A typical lighting programme as used in controlled-environment houses is shown in Table 6.1. Further light stimulation beyond 15 hours can be given if production is not satisfactory. There is rarely any benefit in exceeding 17 hours.

Table 6.1 Typical lighting programme for breeders in controlled-environment housing (from Ross Manual, 1988)

Age		Daylength
Weeks	Days	Hours of light
	1	23
	3	19
	4	16
	5	14
	6	12
	7	11
	8	10
	9	9
	10 to 132	8
19	133	11
20	140	11
21	147	12
22	154	12
23	161	13
24	168	13
25	175	14
26	182	14
27	189	15

However, with all these light programmes it is essential to follow certain basic rules:

1. During periods when the birds are able to respond to light stimulation they are not subjected to decreasing day length; i.e. additional light must be given to prevent a day length reduction.
2. When extending the day length, extra light is provided at both the beginning and the end of the natural daylight period to be certain that the intended day length is achieved.
3. Additional light during this period must be 10–30 lx (1–3 foot-candles) to ensure that the birds are influenced by the additional light. This is brighter than lighting used in light-controlled housing, but is necessary

in view of the brightness of the natural daylight to which the birds are also subjected.

Feed control

The greatest challenge in rearing broiler breeders is to maintain a slow but steady growth, so that the birds are at the correct weight and breeding condition at point of lay at 22 weeks of age. Typical growth curves for males and females are shown in Tables 6.2 and 6.3. In this example, for the Cobb breed, it can be seen that the 22-week weights should be 2.9 kg for males and 2.4 kg for females. The principle is the same for other breeds although the weights will differ slightly.

The growth potential of these birds is so great that if given ad lib feed as in broiler houses these weights would be achieved in about 7 weeks! To achieve the target weights, the birds must therefore be fed a restricted ration, which is an accurately weighed amount of feed calculated on the basis of age, sex and whether the weight of the birds is still on target.

Birds must be weighed weekly, usually a sample of at least 5%, to ensure that they are not over- or under-weight. It is essential to achieve even weights and the coefficient of variation (c.v.) is calculated using the formula:

$$\text{c.v. \%} = \frac{\text{Range of weight} \times 100}{\text{Average weight} \times F}$$

where F value = 4.5 for sample of 50
                = 5.02 for sample of 100

A well-reared flock should have a c.v. of less than 8%. It is vital that if feed is being rationed in this way, it must be distributed evenly and quickly to all the birds, as they are hungry and eat it very quickly. Incorrect feed distribution leading to uneven growth with some birds overweight and some underweight is the single most critical factor which can spoil the subsequent performance of that flock.

Colony size

In order to ensure a coefficient of variation of less than 8% it is essential to partition the flock into pens. A square pen is the ideal shape from the point of view of bird behaviour, therefore the pen size is determined by the house width. The acceptable number of pullets per pen is between 1500 and 1800;

Table 6.2 Female broiler breeder bodyweight targets (Cobb breed) (data from the Cobb Breeding Company Ltd)

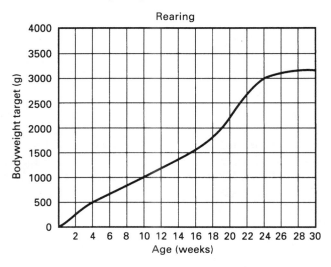

ADULT

Age		Weight		Age		Weight	
weeks	days	g	lb	weeks	days	g	lb
30	210	3180	7.0	45	315	3380	7.5
31	217	3195	7.0	46	322	3390	7.5
32	224	3210	7.1	47	329	3400	7.5
33	231	3225	7.1	48	336	3410	7.5
34	238	3240	7.1	49	343	3420	7.5
35	245	3255	7.2	50	350	3430	7.6
36	252	3270	7.2	51	357	3440	7.6
37	259	3285	7.2	52	364	3450	7.6
38	266	3300	7.3	53	371	3460	7.6
39	273	3315	7.3	54	378	3470	7.6
40	280	3330	7.3	55	385	3480	7.7
41	287	3340	7.4	56	392	3490	7.7
42	294	3350	7.4	57	399	3495	7.7
43	301	3360	7.4	58	406	3500	7.7
44	308	3370	7.4	59	413	3505	7.7
				60	420	3510	7.7

cocks should be housed at 500–1000 per pen. In order to achieve this with houses in excess of 18 m (60 ft) width it will be necessary to construct a centre partition. It is vital that bird numbers are accurately recorded and pen drift is prevented.

The reason for pen separation is to enable the stockperson to identify and separate the light birds. This grading should take place around 5 weeks of age

Table 6.3 Male broiler breeder bodyweight targets (Cobb breed)
(data from the Cobb Breeding Company Ltd)

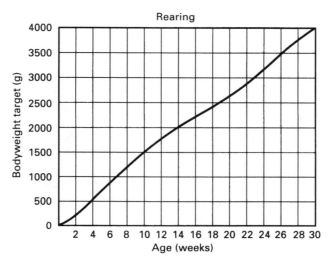

ADULT

Age		Weight		Age		Weight	
weeks	days	g	lb	weeks	days	g	lb
30	210	4010	8.8	45	315	4800	10.6
31	217	4090	9.0	46	322	4820	10.6
32	224	4170	9.2	47	329	4840	10.7
33	231	4235	9.3	48	336	4860	10.7
34	238	4300	9.5	49	343	4880	10.8
35	245	4365	9.6	50	350	4900	10.8
36	252	4430	9.8	51	357	4920	10.8
37	259	4490	9.9	52	364	4940	10.9
38	266	4550	10.0	53	371	4960	10.9
39	273	4600	10.1	54	378	4980	11.0
40	280	4650	10.3	55	385	5000	11.0
41	287	4685	10.3	56	392	5020	11.1
42	294	4720	10.4	57	399	5040	11.1
43	301	4750	10.5	58	406	5060	11.2
44	308	4780	10.5	59	413	5080	11.2
				60	420	5100	11.2

when the 20% lightest birds should be transferred to separate pens which have been left empty for this purpose. After this grading it is important to even up the numbers in the 80% group.

The light birds can now be grown along a growth curve below but parallel to the target weight and from 15 weeks should be gradually brought up to reach the target weight by 21 weeks. If these light birds are not separated they will eventually succumb to the pressures of more aggressive birds and fail to reach point of lay, or if they do survive they will under-perform.

Feed distribution

There are two systems (track and floor) which are normally used for feeding birds during rearing to 18 weeks of age. The daily ration of feed is calculated and weighed out on a beam weighing machine, and held in a hopper on the afternoon before it will be fed. It will then be ready for immediate distribution when the lights come on at around 7.00 a.m. on the next day.

If a trough (track type) feed system is used it is essential that it is of the 'speed feed' type that distributes the feed within about 4 minutes. It is a good idea to cover the tracks with wooden boards until all the feed is distributed. Then remove them at feeding time so that all the birds get an equal chance to eat. About 15 cm (6 in) of feeding space is required for each bird.

The alternative, which has many advantages, is to use floor feeding with pellets. The birds must be introduced to this gradually. First crumbs are provided in chick feeders up to 2 weeks. Then small pellets (2.5×7.0 mm) are given in pans or troughs. At 3 weeks of age, floor feeding can start, putting the feed in lines around the feeders, then at 4 weeks feed is distributed over the total floor area. At 6 weeks the pellet size is increased to 3.2×9.0 mm.

For a floor feeding system to work it is vital that pellets are of good quality, hard and dust free. Litter must be dry and friable. It takes the birds longer to eat their daily ration and they are encouraged to scratch and work the litter, so helping it to stay friable. This also gives the birds exercise.

Water is initially available to birds all the time, but at about 6 weeks it is usual to limit the water availability to approximately 5 hours in the morning and 1 hour in the afternoon. This is done because the birds tend to play with the drinkers, causing spillage, which makes the litter wet; this must be avoided at all costs. It is important to ensure that the level of water in the drinker is no more than about 1 cm to avoid spillage. In hot weather, of course, water may be required for longer periods as it is vital that the birds have sufficient water for their needs.

Transfer to laying house

In most organizations, broiler breeders are reared on one farm to about 18 weeks, and then transferred to the laying farm. This makes better use of facilities and equipment, which are becoming increasingly specialized. Also the people working on the farm become more expert at either 'rearing' or 'laying'. However, the day-old to death system, where the birds remain on the same farm from 0 to 60 weeks, is still used and can be very satisfactory.

On the laying farm, track feeders are generally used with the same requirements for rapid feed distribution in 4 minutes as on the rearing site. Each bird should have 15 cm (6 in) of feeder space. There should be one drinker per 100 birds. Nest boxes should be in place in good time before laying starts, allowing one box per four birds (Plate 6).

At 18 weeks, the males are housed with the females at a ratio of 10 or 11 males per 100 females. When the flock has settled down, this ratio is reduced to 9 males per 100 females. If subsequent mortality in the flock affects a large number of females, it is important that the mating ratio is kept at 9:1, otherwise excessive damage to the pullets may occur through overmating, particularly from 30 weeks onwards. Males should be continually reduced from that time, ensuring a 7% ratio by depletion at 60 weeks.

Feed quantities should be increased each week at this stage. It is becoming common practice to introduce separate sex feeding, with the cockerels being fed from separate hoppers placed out of the reach of the pullets. This stops the cockerels from becoming overweight and therefore helps to maintain fertility as the birds grow older. The male requirement at peak should be in the region of 120 g/bird/day compared to 165–168 g per pullet. A 'toast rack' grid with a critical grid size of 43 mm, is placed on the tracks to allow only pullets to feed from them (Figure 6.1). These may have to be removed at about 50 weeks if birds are becoming too big to eat from them. When this occurs the birds have swollen, puffy faces. This is sometimes mistaken for the disease swollen head syndrome (Duff *et al.* 1989).

It is important to maintain a good atmosphere in the house, without the buildup of ammonia, and to ensure that the litter remains dry and friable. Patches of wet or caked litter should be dug out and removed. Fresh shavings should be added as necessary to keep litter in good condition. Litter and slats are used very successfully in many countries, particularly the USA, where it is the favoured system. The litter should occupy 60% of the floor area, with the slats making up the remaining 40%.

The first eggs should be laid during the 22nd week and peak production will be reached by 30 weeks of age. The weighing of both males and females should continue weekly during lay. Eggs are graded by weight to determine when they will be suitable for hatching, usually at 50 g.

During lay, it is a good practice to weigh a sample of eggs daily as this gives early indication of stresses brought on by disease, nutritional deficiencies, water shortage or temperature extremes.

Feed is distributed automatically on a time clock. It is advisable for this to happen when staff first start work in the morning, so that the birds' feeding

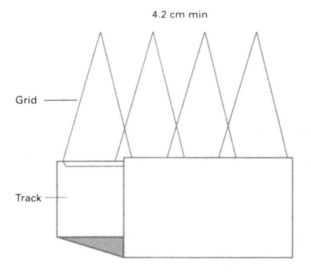

4.2 cm min

Grid

Track

Track guarded by wire grid

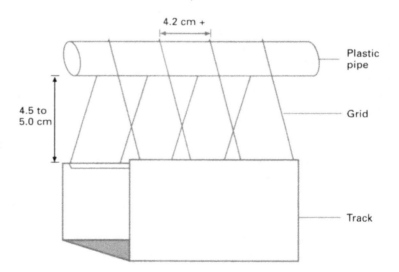

4.2 cm +

Plastic pipe

4.5 to 5.0 cm

Grid

Track

Track guarded by grid and plastic pipe

Figure 6.1 Wire 'toast rack' used on track feeders for broiler breeders.

behaviour can be watched. Although it may be more convenient for the farm staff for feed to be distributed very early so that the eggs are laid and can be collected earlier, they may have missed observing the birds feed, which could be crucial.

In order to ensure pullets do not become progressively fatter, reduction in feed should begin three weeks after the flock has achieved peak production (Table 6.4). Recording of daily egg weights will help to achieve this and feed should only be reduced if the eggs are to target weight.

This is achieved by calculating several parameters based on the following facts. Females achieve sexual maturity at about 23 weeks and physical maturity by 30 weeks. After this time the bird stops growing but will continue to grow fatter, especially if given too much feed. Peak egg production normally occurs at 30 weeks of age and egg mass will peak about 3 weeks later as shown in Figure 6.2. Reduction in daily feed allowances should begin approximately 3 weeks after the flock has achieved peak production.

Eggs should be weighed daily, taking a sample of 150 and excluding double yolks.

$$\text{Egg mass} = \frac{\text{Average egg weight} \times \% \text{ hen day production}}{100}$$

where

$$\text{Hen day production} = \frac{\text{Number of eggs laid in one day}}{\text{Number of hens alive}} \times 100$$

The daily feed reduction will depend on the ambient temperature, nutrient content of feed, flock uniformity and disease status. The figures given in Table 6.4 are thus illustrative only.

Table 6.4 Reduction in feed (g/bird/day) during lay (broiler breeder) (from Ross Manual)

Age (Wks)	Reduction (g/b/d)	Total feed (g/b/d)	Total energy (kcal/b/d)
30		160	440
33	5	155	426
35	3	152	418
37	2	150	412
39	2	148	407
41	1	147	404
43	2	145	399
45	1	144	396
47	2	142	390
49	1	141	388
51	2	139	382
53	1	138	379
55	2	136	374

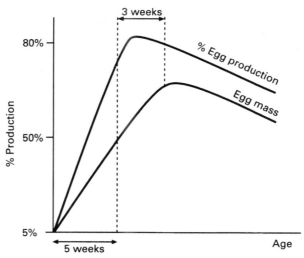

Figure 6.2 Relationship of egg mass to egg production in broiler breeders.

Response to disease

Feed and water restriction have a fundamental effect on the way broiler breeders respond to certain disease conditions and as a result the strategy that needs to be adopted to treat and control them. These restrictions also create a very competitive environment which can result in particularly aggressive behaviour of healthy birds to the sick or less dominant birds.

Under practical conditions of feed restriction, for example, if the level required is 80 g per bird per day, it is assumed that all birds receive 80 g. In fact, this is not so. The flock as a whole receives the correct quantity of feed, so that the average intake of birds in the flock will be 80 g, but some birds will receive more than this and some less. This effect is exacerbated if disease, either clinical or subclinical, is present. With most disease conditions, individual birds are affected at different times and to varying degrees and some may be totally unaffected. This creates a special problem with treatment. In a situation where subclinical disease is present, healthy birds will eat even more than their fair share of the available feed.

Coccidiosis is a good example of a disease which occurs during the rearing period and affects individuals to different degrees. Within one pen, there will often be a range of birds affected from those dying from the disease to those that are totally healthy. Some birds that are only slightly sick will take a little longer to eat their food and may require some encouragement to do so. Unfortunately, the practice of feeding the flock rather than individuals means that the sick bird will not have time to eat sufficient feed causing it to fall further behind the healthy ones. The daily ration of feed is probably consumed by the birds within half an hour, thus the sick birds do not eat their share and the healthy ones eat more than they should. This creates unevenness in body weight and frame size and also means that there is a variable consumption of the coccidiostat in the feed. Unless action is taken fairly quickly to separate small birds from large, the decline in physical condition can become permanent. The long-term effects on the healthy birds that consume more than their share of feed can be as severe as those that suffer disease. If allowed to become too overweight, their future egg production and fertility can be affected. The disease has thus affected both healthy and sick birds adversely.

Medication

Medication rates in broiler breeders should be based on the dose of medication per unit liveweight, as in any other species.

In poultry this is then converted for practical purposes into the dose per tonne of feed or per litre of drinking water. It is this conversion for ease of use that can lead to the incorrect administration of medication in broiler breeders. This is because dosage rates per tonne of feed assumes ad lib feeding, which with broiler breeders is not the case. For example, a 1500–2000 g broiler on ad lib feeding eats approximately 150 g of feed per day. The same weight of broiler breeder, during the rearing stage, could be eating as little as 60 g per day. During lay, a 3.5 kg broiler breeder is rationed to about 160 g per day. Thus the feed intake for a broiler breeder in relation to liveweight is only about half that of a broiler.

There is also another aspect to this situation. If in a broiler house containing 4-week-old birds, individual birds are slightly sick and have depressed appetites, they will take longer to eat their feed than normal. This does not matter because on ad lib feed their daily intake will be virtually normal. Even if they can only eat 70% of normal requirements they have the opportunity to do so. For broiler breeders feed is available for a much shorter time, only 30 minutes per day during rearing and perhaps 1–4 hours per day during lay. Thus a bird with a depressed appetite may have a very low feed consumption and hence the medication rate will be distorted. This may happen, but to a lesser extent with medication in water where water restriction is practised. It would seem logical therefore, to use double the usual medication rate for sick broiler breeders, but this may not entirely solve the problem. If there are many sick birds with depressed appetites, the healthy birds may eat two or three times their daily requirements. Thus they could receive an overdose of medication with a possible risk of toxicity. This could be particularly important with furazolidone and could explain its variable effect on birds in lay.

Thus water medication is the preferred route for treating broiler breeders as the water is available to them for longer periods than feed and also because sick birds will drink more readily than eat and healthy birds will not over-drink. However, for long-term administration of coccidiostats, or for treating chronic disease such as fowl cholera, the feed route is the only practical method of drug administration.

Management of layers

The basic principles of good management already described for broiler breeders apply equally to commercial layers. Thus it is necessary to indicate only the major differences in management practice.

Brooding

Layer chicks may be brooded either on litter on the floor or in cages. The advantages of the cage system is that it gives more effective parasite (mainly coccidiosis) control, savings in feed (providing a good ambient temperature is maintained) and allows a higher stocking density of the building.

Floor system

The equipment needed for brooding 1000 pullets on the floor system is as follows:

- Heating—two gas or radiant heat brooders of 10 000 BTU each.
- Feeding—20 trays.
- Drinkers—10 small fountains or supplementary drinkers.
- Light—1 bulb/brooder.

Brooding continues until approximately 4 weeks of age.
The requirements for 1000 growing pullets are as follows:

- Area—100 m^2 (1000 ft^2).

- Feeding—50 m chain (speed = 1 circuit of the house in 15 minutes) or 50 tube feeders or pans.
- Drinkers—10 large circular drinkers or 10 metres of trough.
- Lighting—450 W (45 lux) for windowed houses; 100 W (10 lux) for windowless houses.

Brooding is usually started at a temperature of 35 °C reducing by about 3 °C every week. In whole-house heating systems, the temperature at day-old is 32 °C reducing by 2–5 °C each week. Post-brooding the ideal temperature is 20 °C. A relative humidity of 75–80% helps to stop dehydration and the onset of pecking.

Cage system

The space requirement per bird is 230 cm^2 (36 in^2) from 0 to 8 weeks and 465 cm^2 (72 in^2) from 8 to 18 weeks. For brooding in cage systems, it is normal to feed on paper or trays for the first five days with one supplementary drinker per cage. The light should be 4 W/m^2 (40 lux). For growing, the birds need 8 cm (3 in) trough space each and a minimum of one nipple for 10 birds for drinking. Lights are reduced to 1 W/m^2 (10 lux).

Feed control

Birds should be weighed weekly, at the same time on the same day prior to feeding. Adjustments can be made if the birds are over or under target (see Chapter 4). For birds in cages, where movement is restricted, environmental temperature is very important. More feed is required to maintain body weight at lower ambient temperatures than at higher temperatures.

Birds will lose weight (8–12% of body weight) when moved to their laying quarters. This loss will take up to five days to regain in controlled-environment housing, but much longer on free range.

Light control

Daylength is reduced gradually from 22 hours at day-old to 8 hours by 8 weeks. Up to 18 weeks, daylength remains on 8 hours and is then gradually increased by 1 hour/week up to 22 weeks. Thereafter it is increased by ½ hour/week to a maximum of 15 hours where it remains to the end of lay. At 17 weeks, the light intensity is increased to 10–15 lux and this level can be maintained throughout lay. Birds usually start to lay at 20 weeks of age.

Ventilation

As with all poultry, it is vital to maintain a good atmosphere in the house with fresh air, free of ammonia. Ventilation requirements depend on house design, insulation and the position of equipment (see Chapter 2). The presence of ammonia will make the birds more susceptible to any respiratory diseases.

Laying period

In cages, the minimum space allowed by welfare codes in the UK is $450\,cm^2/$ bird ($70\,in^2/$bird) with 10 cm (4 in) of trough space per bird and two drinkers (nipples or cups) per cage. On the floor the space allowance is approximately 7 birds/m^2 with 10 cm of trough space allowing one nest for five birds.

Egg production expectations from modern hybrids are enormous. Figure 6.3 shows a typical egg production graph for a brown bird, which is expected to lay 314 eggs (hen housed) from 20 to 80 weeks (assuming an average mortality of 0.12%/week).

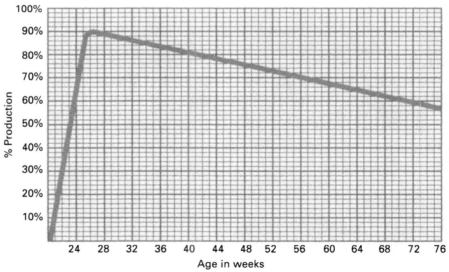

Figure 6.3 Typical egg production graph for commercial layers.

Important diseases of breeders and layers

A number of disease conditions can affect broiler breeders, but in general they have fewer problems than broilers probably because of the much lower stocking density and in general the greater isolation of the farms from other poultry. Layers tend to be housed on sites which are not depopulated (multi-age) so viral respiratory disease, in particular infectious bronchitis, can be a problem. Also many sites are infected with mycoplasma organisms, which can depress overall performance.

Coccidiosis

This is probably the most troublesome condition that occurs in young broiler breeders. A coccidiostat is included in the feed in an attempt to control the disease, without totally eliminating the coccidia. The aim is to allow the coccidia to survive and multiply in the gut of the bird in sufficient numbers to stimulate immunity, which will then be lifelong.

Traditionally, chemical compounds such as amprolium, sulphaquinoxaline and dinitro-o-toluamide have been used for this purpose. However, in recent years the ionophor group of antimicrobial compounds have been found to be more effective. Monensin and salinomycin are both good in this respect. In some situations they are used at a lower dose rate in breeders than in broilers and in a step-down fashion to aid the development of immunity. Thus monensin is used at 60 ppm from 0 to 8 weeks and at 40 ppm from 8 to 16 weeks. This compares with the usual rate of 100 ppm for broilers. However, because of feed restriction the birds are limited in their coccidiostat consumption, as explained above, so it is quite satisfactory to use 100 ppm of monensin or 60 ppm (broiler rate) of salinomycin from 0 to 16 weeks.

Despite the presence of a coccidiostat, the disease may still occur. The most common form is caecal coccidiosis caused by *Eimeria tenella*, which often starts at 4–6 weeks. It usually affects only one pen or one house. There is a sudden but small rise in mortality and dead birds look very pale and anaemic. On post-mortem examination, the characteristic caecal lesions are seen with blood clots and necrotic material causing swollen and enlarged caecae. It is important to start treatment immediately—as the sooner this starts the quicker the recovery. Treatment should be limited to affected houses only. There is no benefit in treating unaffected houses, and in fact this may interfere with the development of coccidial immunity in those birds.

Other forms of intestinal coccidiosis are also seen, caused by *E. necatrix*, *E. brunetti* and *E. maxima*. It is important to have the diagnosis confirmed by a

191

veterinary laboratory as occasionally necrotic enteritis is present in conjunction with coccidiosis.

The usual treatment is to use an amprolium or sulphaquinoxaline preparation in the drinking water. In the cases where necrotic enteritis is present soluble penicillin will be required to control the multiplication of the causal organism, *Clostridium perfringens*.

An outbreak of coccidiosis can be very damaging to the flock, not only in terms of mortality but also in the overall effect on the growth of the birds, causing unevenness in the pen or house. Generally it makes the sorting into large and small birds more difficult and disrupts the feeding programme, as constant adjustments are needed to keep birds on target weight. If the disease could be prevented this would be ideal. Live vaccines in some countries still require the use of drugs for treatment after their administration.

Recently, a vaccine has been developed by workers at Houghton Poultry Research Laboratory from so-called precocious strains of *Eimeria*. Each species of *Eimeria* has been attenuated by growth in fertile eggs to shorten its life cycle. These species have then been combined into a single live vaccine for administration via the drinking water to birds at 5–10 days of age. Now commercially available (Paracox: Pitman-Moore), this vaccine shows great promise.

Staphylococcal infection

Lameness caused by swollen hock joints can be very troublesome in young broiler breeders. At post-mortem when the joints are opened they contain a greyish fluid with yellow flecks, from which pure cultures of *Staphylococcus aureus* can be isolated. Sometimes this pus-like material can be seen to have tracked up the gastrocnemius tendon above the hock joint. This condition usually occurs between 8 and 16 weeks and appears to be associated with the period of maximum feed restriction. Occasionally it is seen in adult birds as well. Affected birds should be culled as they do not respond to treatment, and the rest of the flock treated with a broad-spectrum antibiotic, such as chlortetracycline, in the feed for 2 weeks. It may rarely be seen in adult birds, but should always be distinguished from viral arthritis.

Staphylococcal infection seems to be a bigger problem in track-fed birds where there is fighting and excessive competition for feed. Floor feeding seems to lessen the problem as the birds have more space and are able to exercise more. The provision of perches will help birds to increase their leg strength and it also helps to train them to use nest boxes later on.

The route of infection may be through a break in the skin; this can occur with damage due to poor technique in toe clipping of day-old male chicks, or in the case of adults where wet litter leads to skin cracking of the soles of the feet.

Staphylococcal infection in the feet of adult birds leads to the formation of abscesses, which are hot and painful—a condition known as bumble foot.

Spontaneous tendon rupture

Rupture of the gastrocnemius tendon is sometimes seen in older broiler breeder birds. This may be secondary to infection and inflammation (teno-synovitis) of the tendon sheath caused by staphylococcal infection. However, it can occur spontaneously, when a traumatic aetiology is suggested. Presumably heavier birds are more likely to damage the leg tendons when moving up and down from nest boxes or perches. This form of tendon rupture should always be distinguished from that caused by viral arthritis where the causal agent is a reovirus.

Egg peritonitis

This is a very common cause of mortality as birds come into lay and prior to achieving peak production. Birds bred for meat production have a high ovula-tion rate, so that many more ova are initially produced than are ultimately required for egg production. Some are reabsorbed, but occasionally they are released into the peritoneal cavity and set up infection, which develops into septicaemia.

Post-mortem examination usually reveals yolk debris with large amounts of milky fluid in the abdomen. This usually smells offensive and yields cultures of *Escherichia coli*.

A typical layer or broiler breeder flock may lose up to 1% of birds per month of which a proportion will always be due to egg peritonitis. However, if there is a flock problem with egg peritonitis, mortality can be much higher than this. The cause often relates to faulty management. In broiler breeders it may be due to birds being overweight at point of lay, with excess abdominal fat. In layers it can relate to vent pecking or outbreaks of cannibalism, which are now becoming more common with increasing numbers of free-range flocks.

Marek's disease

After the introduction of a vaccine for Marek's disease for layers and breeders in 1971, the control of this disease was very effective for a number of years. The most commonly used vaccine contains the turkey herpesvirus (THV) and this is given at day old in the hatchery. It is available in either a freeze-dried form or a cell-associated 'wet' vaccine, which is kept in liquid nitrogen. The 'wet' vaccine is considered to be more effective for day-old use. In many countries the challenge from Marek's disease is very high and a second vaccination is required for breeders at 2–3 weeks of age, when usually the freeze-dried THV vaccine is given by intramuscular injection.

There are three different serotypes of Marek's disease virus, so that it is sometimes necessary to use more than one type of vaccine or to use two together (bivalent vaccine) to control field challenge. Serotype 1 vaccine is exemplified by the CVI 988 (Rispens) strain, which is an extremely good vaccine but not permitted in all countries. The SB 1 vaccine is an example of serotype 2 vaccine, and THV is of serotype 3. Often the latter are combined as a single bivalent vaccine. It is a distinct advantage to use one type, say Rispens, at day old followed by THV at 2–3 weeks to give a broader spectrum of protection.

Swollen head syndrome

This is a descriptive term given to a syndrome which has occurred mostly in broiler breeders but also in commercial layers during the last five years (Plates 2 and 8). It is usually seen in laying birds after 30 weeks of age and is characterized by a small drop in egg production, with a variable number of birds showing nervous signs such as torticollis. Affected birds usually have puffy faces with subcutaneous swelling. On post-mortem there is always an acute egg peritonitis, but no other significant lesions. Pure cultures of *Escherichia coli* can be obtained from the peritoneum and most organs, including the meninges and middle ear. Affected birds must be culled as they do not respond to treatment, but the flock as a whole will benefit from treatment in feed with a broad-spectrum antibiotic such as chlortetracycline for 14 days. It has been shown that birds seroconvert to turkey rhinotracheitis virus (Wyeth *et al.* 1987) during the course of this disease and as the syndrome has only been seen since TRT became apparent, it seems that this virus is likely to be the causal agent with *E. coli* a secondary pathogen (Pattison *et al.* 1989).

Fowl cholera

This disease is caused by the bacterium *Pasteurella multocida*. It can be a very severe acute infection with birds in good condition 'found dead on their nests'. More commonly, it causes a chronic infection with low mortality which affects egg production and causes swollen wattles. The infection is carried into poultry houses by wild birds or rodents (especially rats) and spreads between birds via the drinking water. The infection can only be removed from the site by an extremely thorough clean out and disinfection at the end of the life of the flock. If a site has been infected it is wise to vaccinate the next flock using two doses of a killed vaccine given at 8 and 12 weeks of age. If this flock then remains unaffected, it should be possible to rear the next flock on that site without vaccination.

In affected flocks, the use of broad-spectrum antibiotics such as tetracyclines gives useful control. Initial medication for about five days in the water is followed by more prolonged treatment in the feed.

Pasteurellae can be a cause of lameness in young birds, where the swelling of the hock joints looks like a staphylococcal infection. The two conditions can only be distinguished by bacterial culture.

Fowl coryza

This disease is caused by the bacterium *Haemophilus paragallinarum* and is a problem in certain countries only. Affected birds show depression, with nasal discharge, conjunctivitis and facial swelling. Diagnosis must be confirmed by isolating the causal organism. The disease is usually more severe if other respiratory viral infections are present and it is usually introduced to a farm by infected stock. The use of killed vaccine by injection at 16–18 weeks of age usually controls the disease.

Chick anaemia virus

The importance of immunity to this viral infection has only recently been understood. A serological survey of breeding flocks in the UK (McNulty *et al.* 1988) showed the presence of antibody to be widespread. However, there is a trend now to increase the level of hygiene and the degree of isolation in breeder flocks in an attempt to eradicate salmonella infection as happened in Sweden some years ago. This may lead to some flocks not being exposed to the chick anaemia virus. If a flock is still susceptible to infection during lay and then is exposed to virus, it will transmit virus to the progeny through the egg until immunity develops. This period of virus excretion causes the development of 'blue wing' disease in infected chicks between 2 and 4 weeks of age. This is a form of gangrenous dermatitis affecting the wing tips and the chicks show lymphoid depletion with anaemia. Mortality is often considerable. In some countries it may be necessary to vaccinate breeders if natural exposure does not occur. A suitable vaccine (TAD Thymus Vac. manufactured by Lohman) has recently been developed and is licensed for use in some countries.

Infectious bursal disease (IBD)

This disease was originally called Gumboro disease after the town in North America where it was first described. It is a viral disease which formerly caused mortality only in broilers. However, since the appearance of a virulent strain in Europe in 1987, it is now an important disease of layers and occasionally also breeders. The first sign of this disease is usually a rise in mortality, which lasts about five days. Post-mortem lesions are diagnostic and consist of swelling of the bursa of Fabricius and haemorrhages in skeletal muscle of the thighs and breast.

Control is only possible by a combination of hygiene including thorough cleaning between crops and vaccination. To control this extremely virulent form of the disease, three or four doses of the live intermediate strain of vaccine may be required. In layer replacements, killed vaccine has also been used successfully with the vaccine given by injection during the first week of life.

Monitoring and vaccination programmes

The value of breeding and laying stock and the fact that they will live for about 1 year means that it is essential to have an efficient system of monitoring and vaccination. The recent requirement in the UK for salmonella testing of breeding and laying flocks has reinforced this need for a monitoring programme. Vaccinations required will vary in different countries and different areas, but usually stock should have protection from Marek's disease, Newcastle disease, infectious bronchitis, infectious bursal disease, infectious avian encephalomyelitis and egg drop syndrome. Fowl pox and infectious laryngotracheitis and reovirus protection is also required in some situations. Veterinary advice should always be taken before deciding which vaccines are required and in what order they should be given. Some examples are shown in Tables 6.5–6.8.

Vaccines for poultry are available in two forms, live and killed. Live vaccines consist of living organisms which have been modified (attenuated) so that they will multiply in the host without causing disease. They can be given in a variety of ways—via the drinking water, coarse spray, eye drop or in the case of Marek's disease by intramuscular injection. The development of immunity is more rapid with live vaccines than with killed ones. Killed vaccines consist of inactivated (dead) organisms which are usually suspended in an oily emulsion for administration by injection. The emulsion helps to promote an even more prolonged uptake of the organisms from the site of inoculation. Full immunity develops about one month after injection of the killed vaccine. The ideal method of vaccination is to give a live vaccine first, which acts as a 'primer' for the immune system, followed by the injection of killed vaccine, which gives a sustained level of protective antibody. This principle applies to

Table 6.5 Vaccination programme—Far East

Age	Vaccine	Route
1 day	Marek's disease	Intramuscular
	Infectious bronchitis H120	Intra-ocular
7 days	Newcastle disease B1	Intra-ocular
10 days	Coccivac	Drinking water
2 weeks	Infectious bursal disease	Drinking water
3 weeks	Newcastle disease, LaSota	Intra-ocular
	Infectious bronchitis H120	Intra-ocular
	Fowl pox	Wing web
6 weeks	Coryza	Intramuscular
7 weeks	Infectious bursal disease	Drinking water
8 weeks	Newcastle disease, LaSota	Intra-ocular
	Newcastle disease, killed	Subcutaneous
14 weeks	Avian encephalomyelitis and	Wing web
	Fowl pox	
16 weeks	Coryza and egg drop syndrome	Intramuscular
20 weeks	Infectious bronchitis,	
	Newcastle disease,	Subcutaneous
	Infectious bursal disease, killed	
38 weeks	Newcastle disease, LaSota	Intra-ocular
	Newcastle disease, killed	Subcutaneous
48 weeks	Newcastle disease, LaSota	Intra-ocular
	Newcastle disease, killed	Subcutaneous

protection against Newcastle disease, infectious bronchitis and infectious bursal disease. For each of these a more attenuated (milder) live vaccine is generally used first followed by a less attenuated (stronger) vaccine, which can be used in the programme before the killed vaccine.

For Newcastle disease, the mild vaccine used first is called the B1 strain and this can be followed by the LaSota strain. The LaSota strain is essential in countries where Newcastle disease is enzootic, but it is not permitted in the UK, where Newcastle disease has been eradicated. This is sensible as in fully susceptible birds the LaSota virus is able to multiply and spread amongst a flock of birds causing respiratory disease in its own right.

Two types of live vaccine are available for infectious bronchitis, the H_{120} mild strain and the H_{52} which is more attenuated. H_{120} must always be used first as H_{52} will produce disease in unprimed birds. In some countries 'variant' strains of live IB vaccines are also needed for priming.

For infectious bursal disease a variety of live vaccines are available, which

Table 6.6 Vaccination programme—South America

Age	Vaccine	Route
1 day	Marek's disease	Intramuscular
14 days	Fowl pox	Wing web
	Newcastle disease B1	Drinking water
	Infectious bronchitis H120	Drinking water
	Marek's disease	Intramuscular
4 weeks	Infectious bursal disease	Drinking water
	Newcastle disease, LaSota	Drinking water
8 weeks	Fowl cholera	Subcutaneous
	Newcastle disease, LaSota	Intra-ocular
	Infectious bronchitis H120	Drinking water
10 weeks	Infectious laryngotracheitis	Intra-ocular
12 weeks	Avian encephalomyelitis/Fowl pox	Wing web
	Fowl cholera	Subcutaneous
	Newcastle disease, LaSota	Intra-ocular
14 weeks	Coryza	Intramuscular
16 weeks	Egg drop syndrome	Intramuscular
18 weeks	Coryza	
	Newcastle disease	
	Infectious bronchitis	Intramuscular
	Infectious bursal disease	
35 weeks	Newcastle disease, LaSota	Spray
	Infectious bronchitis H120	

Table 6.7 Vaccination programme for broiler and layer breeders in the UK

Age	Vaccine	Route
1 day	Marek's disease	Intramuscular
2 weeks	Marek's disease	Intramuscular
3 weeks	Newcastle disease B1	
	Infectious bronchitis H120 and	Drinking water
	Infectious bursal disease	
8 weeks	Newcastle disease B1	Drinking water or spray
	Infectious bronchitis H120	Drinking water or spray
10 weeks	Infectious bursal disease	Drinking water
14 weeks	Avian encephalomyelitis	Drinking water
16 weeks	Newcastle disease	
	Infectious bronchitis (Mass.)	Intramuscular
	Infectious bursal disease	

Table 6.8 Vaccination programme for commercial egg layers in the UK

Age	Vaccine	Route
1 day	Marek's disease	Intramuscular
	Infectious bursal disease	Spray/injection
3 weeks	Newcastle disease B1	Drinking water or spray
	Infectious bronchitis H120 and	
	Infectious bursal disease	Drinking water
7 weeks	Newcastle disease B1	
	Infectious bronchitis H120 and	Drinking water
	Infectious bursal disease	
10 weeks	Avian encephalomyelitis	Drinking water
14 weeks	Infectious bronchitis	
	Newcastle disease	Intramuscular
	Egg drop syndrome	

vary from mild through intermediate to hot strains. It is essential to use only the mild or intermediate strains for priming.

Protection against infectious avian encephalomyelitis (epidemic tremor) requires only one dose of the live vaccine for lifelong immunity in breeders and layers.

In the case of fowl cholera, coryza and egg drop syndrome only dead vaccines are available.

The live vaccine for fowl pox must be given, as with all poxvirus vaccinations, by skin scarification. In chickens the most convenient site for this is the wing web. Infectious laryngotracheitis vaccine is a potentially 'hot' strain and should only be used in areas where the disease is enzootic. It is usually given by eye drop.

Killed vaccines are usually given by deep muscle injection in the thigh or breast muscle, but some such as fowl cholera (pasteurella) vaccine are usually given under the skin at the back of the neck (Plate 7). The vaccinations carried out should be recorded on a chart and kept as a permanent record on the farm, showing the batch number of vaccine, the date vaccination was carried out, and the name of the person who carried out the vaccination. If birds are moved from rearing to laying quarters, the record should go with them.

Birds should receive two doses of piperazine worm powder in drinking water at 14 and 16 weeks of age, with a third dose if necessary at 22 weeks. This should be sufficient to control *Ascaris* sp., the large roundworm of poultry, which is always present to a greater or lesser degree. Occasionally, *Capillaria* may be a problem, in which case a different wormer will be required such as fenbendazole, given in feed for one week at around 16 weeks of age. In countries where tapeworms are a problem, birds should be routinely treated with a suitable wormer.

Salmonella testing

For many years, primary breeding companies have carried out intensive testing programmes for *Salmonella* spp. to ensure freedom from the egg-transmitted types. *S. pullorum* and *S. gallinarum* have been eradicated for many years in most poultry enterprises, so now it is important to check for the less poultry-specific types such as *S. typhimurium* and *S. enteritidis*. Routine monitoring of parent stock and layers is now a legal requirement in the UK and follows a similar programme to that used by the more responsible companies for many years (Breeding and Hatcheries Order, Layers Order (1989)).

Routine blood testing

It is routine practice to check the level of antibody (titre) to the main diseases covered in the vaccination programme. This is a check to ensure that the vaccinations have been carried out properly and also gives a baseline from which to work, should some subsequent disease problem occur. It is necessary to take at least 20 samples from each house and it is a good idea to sample immediately prior to giving killed vaccine, i.e. at about 16 weeks and then 4–6 weeks later at 20–22 weeks, to check the response to killed vaccines and again after peak egg production at 32 weeks. The results of these blood tests should be kept with the flock records so that they are available for investigation of any later problems. The enzyme-linked immunosorbent assay (ELISA) blood testing system is particularly useful in this regard as large numbers of sample results can be stored on computer discs and results between and within flocks easily compared for all the different diseases. It is usual to measure titres for Newcastle disease, infectious bronchitis, infectious bursal disease, and perhaps in some situations infectious avian encephalomyelitis and egg drop syndrome. A number of commercially available kits are now available for carrying out ELISA testing.

Figures 6.4 and 6.5 show examples of ELISA tests displayed in histogram form. The name of the farm, age of birds, assay being carried out and the titre are all shown. There is also a column for remarks.

Investigating a drop in egg production

One of the most common problems in breeders and layers is investigating the cause of a fall in egg production. A checklist should be prepared to enable the investigator, whether stockperson or veterinarian, to cover all the possibilities in a logical order. The main points that should be checked are as follows:

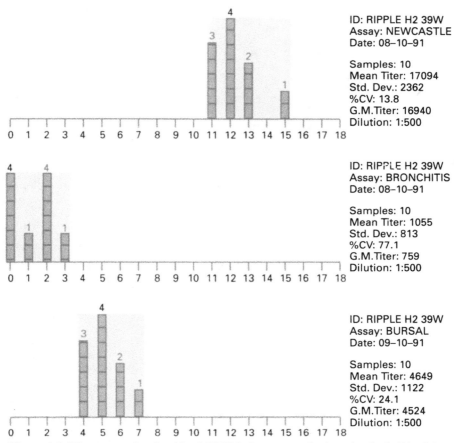

Figure 6.4 Histograms showing blood ELISA titre groups for breeder flock (Ripple), age 39 weeks.

1. Water consumption—has there been a sudden interruption to the supply? Check water meters, if fitted, in each house. A water sample should be taken if there is any possibility of contamination.
2. Does the drop in production coincide with a new feed delivery and if so has this batch of feed been distributed to the bins in all the houses? A feed sample should be taken from current feed batches.
3. Have there been any power cuts? Check the setting on time clocks to ensure that lights are coming on and going off when they are supposed to. Ventilation should be checked to see if it is working correctly.
4. Do the birds look healthy? If not, are there any signs of disease or a rise in mortality?
5. Are the eggs normal in size and shape? If not, are there soft shells or

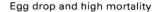

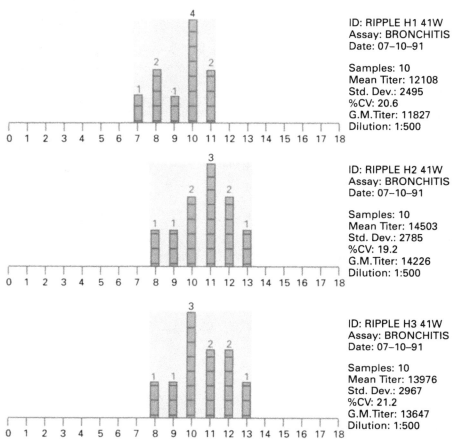

Figure 6.5 Blood test results in flock 'Ripple' after a drop in egg production due to infectious bronchitis in three different houses, H_1, H_2 and H_3.

signs of excess calcification? Is there a rise in the number of seconds at the packing station?

6. Has there been any change in management or staff looking after the birds? Also have there been any visitors who could have frightened the birds, e.g. a vaccination team?

7. Is stocking density on the floor or in cages appropriate to the breed and climate?

8. Check point-of-lay body weights and rearing history with vaccination records.

9. Take a selection of organs to store in the deep freeze for later virus isolation if necessary. For example trachea, gut contents, caecal tonsils,

SVH Ripple Mean I.B. Titre @ 18 w, 23 w, 31 w, 39 w, and 41 w

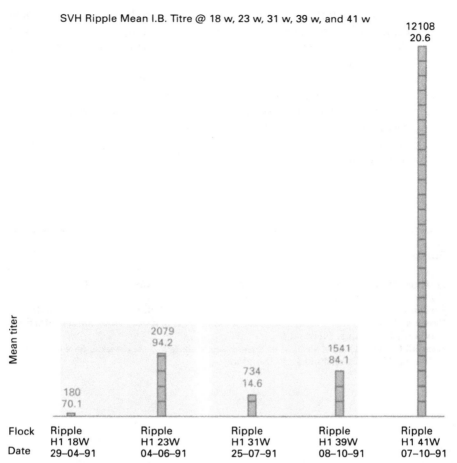

Figure 6.6 Sequential blood test results for flock 'Ripple' from 18 weeks showing sudden rise in infectious bronchitis titre.

spleen and liver are usually sufficient. Also keep tissues in 10% formol saline for histology if required later.

10. It is wise to take blood samples immediately from affected houses. The sera can be stored if not required for immediate testing. If the problem has not been resolved, another set of samples should be taken from the same houses and tested for infectious disease. 'Paired' serum samples taken in this way, enable the diagnostician to see if the titre to any infectious disease has risen during the time when the problem existed. (See Figure 6.6 where there was a rise in titre to IB infection between 39 and 41 weeks and also the virus was isolated from caecal tonsils and gut contents.)

Possible infectious causes of a drop in egg production are: Newcastle disease/influenza; infectious bronchitis; egg drop syndrome; turkey rhinotracheitis (swollen head syndrome); infectious laryngotracheitis; and fowl cholera.

Feed should be checked for any major abnormality initially to ensure it is the correct feed, i.e. layer or breeder feed. Check protein, oil and calcium. A manganese assay will determine whether the supplement was added. Other compounding errors are possible, such as the accidental inclusion of nicarbazine or ionophor coccidiostats and these should be tested for if appropriate.

Further reading

Hofstad M S, Barns H J, Calnek B W, Reid W M, Yoder H W Jr. (eds) (1991) *Diseases of poultry.* Iowa State College Press, Ames, Iowa.

Jordan F T W (ed) (1990) *Poultry diseases.* 3rd edition. Baillière Tindal, London.

Payne L N (ed) (1985) *Marek's diseases: scientific basis and methods of control.* Martinus Nijhoff Publishing, New York.

Randall C J (1991) *A colour atlas of diseases and disorders of the domestic fowl and turkey.* 2nd ed. Wolfe Publishing Ltd., London.

DISEASE PREVENTION AND CONTROL IN TURKEYS
J C STUART BVSc, MRCVS, DPMP

Introduction
The modern industry
Rearing methods and commercial fattening
Breeder management
Disease prevention
Important diseases of turkeys
Further reading

Introduction

The modern turkey originated from the wild turkey of Central and North America where it was an important source of food for the American Indians. The Red Indian chief had rare eagle feathers in his head-dress. The braves had turkey feathers! His arrows were tipped with the sharp turkey spurs and fletched with the stiff wing feathers.

Columbus mistook them for peacocks. His men called them 'Toka', the Tamil name for a peacock. Later this was converted into the Hebrew 'Tukki' by the Jewish merchants in Spain, and still later anglicized to 'Turkey'. Nothing whatsoever to do with the country of that name!

Benjamin Franklin wrote to his daughter: 'I wish the bald eagle had not been chosen as a representative of our country—the turkey is a much more respectable bird, and a true original native of America.' In the 16th century, wild turkeys were brought over to Spain from Central America, and spread through Europe to England. Improved domesticated strains went back to New England with the early settlers in the 17th century. Even better strains were taken by an English breeder, Jessie Throessel, to British Columbia in 1920. The modern bird was developed from these, along the West Coast of America.

Daniel Defoe in his book *A Tour of England and Wales* in 1724 wrote about some 300 droves of turkeys, varying in size from 100 to 1000 birds, going to London via Ipswich, Sudbury and Clare, each September and October. He reckoned that 15 000 turkeys travelled this way—a slow job. Wealthier farmers later had carts divided into four sections, one above the other, which would only take two days and two nights with a change of horses to reach London.

The original turkey was a small blackish-brown bird that by selective breeding has been changed into the present broad, dimple breasted, white bird with shorter legs and neck. There are still some Norfolk Blacks in existence, and a few bronze and lilac birds on rare breed farms.

The modern industry

A few major breeders supply most of the turkeys reared throughout the world—British United Turkeys, Nicholas and Hybrid Turkeys are all owned by large pharmaceutical or international conglomerates. A plethora of smaller breeders supply specialized markets. Approximately 36 million turkey poults are produced by the British turkey industry in a year, with some 400 million world-wide, mainly from France, Italy, Israel and the USA.

The degree of integration is exemplified by the UK, where four companies produce 75% of the birds. These companies are in production all the year round. Most are fully integrated with their own parent breeding stock, hatcheries, fattening sites, mills, processing plants and sales force. Turkey meat is said to be the most economical source of meat protein commercially available. It is also low in fat—10% compared with 24% in beef and 23% in pork.

Rearing methods and commercial fattening

Details of rearing vary from company to company. Most of the birds are reared and fattened in the same house environment, with males and females kept in separate pens. The females are killed at 10–16 weeks (3.6–6.4 kg, 8–14 lb), which leaves room in the houses for the stags to grow until they are killed at 16–22 weeks (6.8–14.5 kg, 15–32 lb). The killing weight is influenced by the strain of bird, the feeding regimes and the health status; the genetic potential for this weight is increasing by 3% each year. At day old the birds have 930 cm^2 (1 ft^2) per bird while the stags finish off at 2800 cm^2 (3 ft^2) per bird.

Other producers rear in brooder houses until 6 weeks in the summer or 8 weeks in the winter and then move out to pole barns. These are mainly producers who sell New York dressed birds or dry-plucked chilled birds. It requires less capital expense and is said to produce a better finished bird. On the other hand the bird requires more room—4650 cm^2 (5 ft^2) per stag—eats more food, takes longer to reach the required weight and needs more frequent littering. It is essential that the roofs are insulated to prevent condensation. This is an expanding 'green' market.

A few people still use tier brooding cages for the first three weeks. Range rearing is a thing of the past in the UK, but is used extensively in the USA. There is a lot of food wastage and many problems with disease, predators and labour. However, recently there has developed a small specialist market for free-range birds.

The brooding period is the most difficult part of a turkey's life. Day-old poults are partially blind and have well-developed suicidal tendencies. They must be surrounded by heat, light, water and food otherwise they do not start to eat and drink and as a result die in large numbers by the 5th–7th day of age once the yolk sac has been absorbed. The day-olds are therefore placed in a preheated, fully prepared house on clean shavings with all the drinkers and feeders in position. They should be given spot heat of 35 °C (95 °F) and a house heat of 24 °C (75 °F) reducing by 2 °C a week after the first week to 18–20 °C (65–70 °F) by 5 weeks old and held at that until slaughter of the hens. Stags are fattened at a lower temperature of 12–15 °C if possible which produces better feather cover, reduces leg problems and increases the percentage of white meat on the carcase.

Turkeys do not like whole house heating. More poults are lost or damaged through overheating than chilling. They need a variation in temperature and humidity to mimic the natural 'broody hen'. Chilled birds are prone to digestive problems and pasted vents, overheated birds to kidney damage, dehydration, visceral gout and vent pecking.

When birds are going to be reared in pole barns they should be off heat by 5 weeks except for some at night if weather conditions are very cold—otherwise they become 'hooked on heat' and soon create problems by huddling when the heat is finally removed.

Most brooders are designed for chicks—it is usual to put 500 poults under a 1000 chick brooder. Overcrowding causes major losses. Obviously, the brooders have to be well maintained.

The position of the poults tells the stockperson about their state of comfort: if they are too hot the poults will be spread around the edge of the surrounds panting; if too cold they will be huddled under the brooder; if they feel a draught they will all be to one side of the pen. The noise they make also indicates if they are comfortable. Thermometers act as a guide for setting up the house, *not* for day-to-day running.

The houses should have concrete floors and entrances. All sorts of litters have been tried as alternatives to shavings, which are expensive and can be scarce: chopped straw or hay may cake and carry the risk of *Aspergillus* infection; shredded paper initially cakes then becomes very dusty; bark is very dusty. A higher light intensity is required with all of these. Re-used litter produces ammonia problems. If available, shavings are the best, littered to

10 cm (4 in) deep. If house temperature and ventilation are controlled effectively less litter is required initially. More is then added as necessary. Turkeys do not scratch the litter like chickens and so only utilize the top layer.

The poults are kept under the brooders by surrounds of cardboard or wire, which are slowly enlarged until finally they are removed at 7–10 days. Some people place cardboard on the floors of the surrounds to stop litter eating and gizzard impaction. This is not necessary if the environment is set up correctly. Some small flint grit is spread on the food from the second day. However, this can be overdone—the birds may fill themselves with grit and die of starvation.

The numbers of feeding trays (three per 100 poults) and water points (two per 100) are gradually reduced from 10 days onwards, leaving one tube or pan feeder/40 birds, and one drinker/150 birds though some people use less than these—one drinker to 250 and 6–8 tube feeders per 1000 birds. Chain feeders are not suitable for turkeys.

It is very important that any changes in house furniture are made gradually. Turkeys are very stupid. Some will die from kidney failure or dehydration rather than drink from a different drinker, if these are not gradually introduced into the house. The best-run houses have all the final drinkers and feeders in use from day 1 to avoid undue stress.

When young, the birds follow the stockperson and crowd up against the brooding surrounds, with the risk of suffocation. The stockperson, having checked that the house and the birds are alright after placing, should then leave them alone for at least 12 hours to allow them to settle.

As the birds grow the lip of the feeders and drinkers should be continually raised just above the level of the bird's back to avoid food and water spillage and deteriorating litter. Initially there should be plenty of water in the drinkers. By 3 weeks the level should have been decreased to avoid spillage, but not so much that the birds have to tilt the drinkers to drink. Shavings must not be allowed to collect in the feeders, especially not in the feed trays during the first few days. This can be a cause of 'starve outs' or poor uneven flocks.

Starter rations contain 29% protein and 11.7 MJ/kg (2795 kcal/kg) metabolizable energy; these are gradually changed over the growing period to 14.0% protein and 12.89 MJ/kg (3080 kcal/kg) ME. In hot weather, because of the reduced feed consumption, the protein, vitamin and mineral levels are increased by approximately 12%. Reduced levels in the early rations can create leg problems.

Light

Various light patterns are in use. Basically the birds must initially have bright light under the brooders and in the surrounds—100 W for 48 hours providing continuous illumination of the feeders and drinkers without any shadows.

Thereafter, from days 2 to 4, 18 hours, 15 W under and 100 W over the brooder. By 4 weeks old the light intensity of the house should be low—15 W with a daylength of 8 hours, just bright enough to allow them to eat. Some breeds, however, will not tolerate these low light intensities. When birds are subjected to this routine they do not need beak trimming. If the birds are not trimmed and not kept in dim light they start to peck and destroy each other from about the 10th day. Vent pecking occurs if it is too warm, too humid or if the young poults are chilled. Feather pecking occurs as they develop feathers and start to strut in bright light. Where longer periods of bright light are maintained the poults have to be beak trimmed.

Birds going into pole barns and future breeders have to be beak trimmed. Beak trimming is done at day old in the hatchery, or 5–10 days old, or 4 weeks old. Great care is necessary to prevent fatalities occurring due to birds bleeding to death, birds not being able to eat, burnt tongue or respiratory problems due to damaged nostrils. The upper beak is cut or burnt by one-third of its length to just in front of the nostrils, and the lower beak tipped. The depths of food and water available should be increased for a few days for the older birds.

Ventilation

High-speed ventilation is now in vogue, whereby a stream of fresh air is drawn rapidly over the ceiling collecting foul air and losing some fresh air on its way from the inlet to the outlet. It therefore provides a good even atmosphere that is essential for efficient turkey rearing. There should be a minimum of $2\,m^3$ air per second per tonne of feed consumed per day and a maximum of $20\,m^3$ air per second per tonne of feed consumed per day. The minimum rate will have to be increased if ammonia levels increase. Air inlet space must be increased in line with increased fan speeds. Horizontal turbulence fans adjusted to blow diagonally across a house but not onto the birds, are useful after about 7 weeks of age in maintaining the even atmosphere. After brooding, ventilation is the next most difficult thing to control. This is not surprising when one considers the different designs of houses that are used.

Good ventilation and maintenance of house warmth are essential for the well-being of the birds, and there is a very fine balance between the two. This was especially so when the turkeys were infected with *Mycoplasma gallisepti-cum*, when some heat had to be sacrificed in order to effect better ventilation. One must never sacrifice ventilation in an attempt to maintain house temperature. If the litter becomes wet or caked due to inadequate ventilation, water spillage or diarrhoea, foot, leg and breast blister problems develop. Turkeys do not scratch and work the litter like chickens.

Breeder management

Breeders are reared in exactly the same way as the fatteners though they are usually given more space. Hens should be allocated 1400 cm^2 (1.5 ft^2) and stags 2800 cm^2 (3 ft^2) at day old, increasing to 6000 cm^2 (6.5 ft^2) for hens in lay and 9300 cm^2 (10 ft^2) for adult stags. They should be reared in all-in/all-out single-aged sites.

In some countries continuous production stag farms are being used. These have many disadvantages as well as advantages.

All breeding stock are beak trimmed and many are de-snooded. They are carefully selected for conformation and weight throughout the rearing period. The weight of the breeder at the age at which its progeny are to be slaughtered is very important, more so than that at point of lay. One stag is kept per eight hens selected, although this is variable from operation to operation and depends a lot on whether an extender-diluent is used with the semen for artificial insemination (AI).

The optimum age of start of lay for the turkey is between 32 and 34 weeks of age. If she is brought into lay earlier than this there will be more small eggs and fewer eggs in total. If laying starts later, fewer often larger eggs are laid, which may cause increased problems with prolapses.

Light programme

The most important factor influencing egg production is the lighting pattern that the turkey hen receives. Prior to 18 weeks the hen's development is not influenced by daylength. At 18 weeks she should have 7 hours light. This conditioning short daylength is essential for optimum production. A common mistake is to put the hen onto this short daylength too late. If exposure to short daylengths is delayed until she has started to respond to light as shown by squatting, subsequent production will be harmed. Special dark houses are used which should be fully lightproof, with no daylight entering through cracks or fan boxes. These are necessary for flocks maturing during the spring or summer months. At other times of the year, the natural daylength is satisfactory.

Unless she is receiving more than 10 hours light, the turkey hen will not commence lay, regardless of her age. To achieve the best and most uniform results the daylength should be increased in one step to 14–15 hours light at 29.5 weeks, three weeks before eggs are required. This is usually done by moving the birds into open-sided laying houses, though controlled-environment houses are being used more and more. An intensity of at least 70 lx is required for optimum production. If the daylength is increased gradually, there is a spread in the onset of lay by individual birds and poorer results overall are obtained. The surest indication that something is wrong with the pre-lay management is a slow rise to peak and a lower peak in the characteristic egg production curve. The birds respond best to a wavelength of 650 nm (red light), least of all to wavelengths above 700 nm or below 550 nm (green light). Blue fluorescent lights must be avoided. They are most sensitive to light stimulus about 12 hours after the lights come on, so dark afternoons must be avoided by providing supplementary sources of light.

Management in lay

The breeding ration is introduced at the time of moving into the laying quarters.

At the start of lay, it is the turkey's natural instinct to look for a suitable nesting site. Each flock should, therefore, have a sufficient number of nests. There should be one nest box for every four hens in the flock (Plate 11). Many nest boxes have a trap nest front to prevent more than one hen entering the nest at a time. These should be tied open for the first few days of lay to allow the hens to get used to the nest boxes. In some companies, smaller nest boxes are used in which the hen cannot turn round nor can other hens get into the nest. Automatic rollaway nests have been introduced with variable results. In many cases, the birds do not like them and will not use them.

Any hen sitting in dark corners should be caught and placed in a nest to show her the proper place to lay. This can be very laborious. All dark corners in the house should be eliminated. They should not be created by stacking straw bales against the walls. Any hen that is acting unnaturally, is agitated or walking up and down the sides of the pen, is thinking about laying and should be placed in a nest box. The success of these management aspects is shown by the number of floor eggs; these should account for less than 1% of all eggs laid. If the hen persists in laying on the floor in the dark, she will go broody without being noticed. A critical period is reached in the third week of lay, earlier in some breeds, when some hens will commence to go broody, although this tendency has been considerably reduced in the modern breeds of turkey. The egg production graph can once again tell a great deal. The flock will reach its normal peak of egg production around the third week of lay.

Broody management

If no action is taken over hens showing signs of going broody, they will go completely out of lay and production will fall sharply to the level of that of the non-broody hens. Broodiness is exhibited most in hot weather. With the very best management, the hens going broody are spotted before they are fully broody, so that there is only a pause of a few days in egg production. The better the broody control, the smoother will be the egg production curve (Plate 12).

The turkey hen uses the same nest box continually. If she is moved to another pen, it is equivalent to making her desert her old nest to recommence a new clutch of eggs. So judging the time when many of the birds in the flock are on the verge of broodiness is most important. The flock may then be switched to a different pen or house with a different layout of furniture and, if in a pole barn, with the sun entering the house from a different direction. The skill lies in judging the best time to switch the flock.

The onset of broodiness is preceded by a longer time being spent on the nest. The manager's best guide to the timing of a switch is when the nests appear to be getting fuller in the evening. Most eggs are laid at midday. However, flocks should not be switched before peak production is reached in the third week, neither should they be switched more frequently than three-weekly intervals. It is better if this interval can be increased following each switch of pens, since each move is accompanied by a slight loss in egg production. In some organizations some flocks are not moved at all.

Regular daily individual broody inspections must be made, preferably first thing in the morning. In one very effective system, at the end of the day the stockperson drives all the birds on the floor in front of the nests into the main pen area. Those hens on the nest are there for one of two purposes, either to lay or to go broody. The gates or the net dividing the main floor area from the nest are closed, leaving all hens on the nest. This nest area is not more than one-third of the total floor area. In the morning, those hens laying an egg will be off the nest on the floor. Those left on the nest are the broodies which are caught and put in a broody pen for 3 days. Another routine to aid broody control is to push all hens off the nest at each egg collection—six times a day.

Artificial insemination (Plate 9)

There is no natural mating with the modern turkey. The hens are artificially inseminated (AI) twice at 3-day intervals during the 10 days prior to point of lay, as soon as 90% start to squat and can be 'split' i.e. the opening of the oviduct exposed (Plate 10). The utero-vaginal glands must be filled with sperm before the bird starts to lay. A third insemination is given 7 days after the second insemination and thereafter every 7–10 days; usually the older the flock the more frequent the insemination. Fertile eggs may be produced for 18–24 days after insemination.

Stag management

Stags are penned in small groups, fed a different ration (low calcium and phosphorus levels) and must be given an increased daylength (12 hours) 6 weeks before they are required to produce semen. Some stags react to increased daylengths by developing a paralysis of the neck. They do not need a period of short daylength like the hens, but have the same period of daily photosensitivity 12 hours after the lights come on. They are kept on a lower light intensity (5–10 lx; 0.5–1 foot-candle) than the hens to encourage persistent semen production of good quality. Some organizations restrict the amount of food given to the stags to prevent them putting on too much weight and developing leg problems.

The stags are milked (stimulated to produce semen) up to three times a week and have to be trained to ejaculate before the hens require insemination. Each hen is inseminated with 0.01–0.03 ml of bulked semen from several stags by deep insemination (5 cm; 2 in) using a different tube for each hen.

Semen is held at 15 °C (59 °F) for not more than 30 minutes. A diluent is frequently used, reducing the amount of semen and hence the number of stags required.

Breed standards

Birds are kept in lay for 18–22 weeks. The number of settable eggs and poults expected in a 24-week laying period varies with the breed of the bird; typical average figures are:

BUT 8	112 settable eggs	→ 92 poults
Nicholas	100 settable eggs	→ 79 poults
Hybrid	97 settable eggs	→ 76 poults

In general, the genetic potential for egg production is increasing by one egg per year. Heavy breeds produce fewer eggs than lighter breeds.

It must be remembered that for birds to perform identically they must have identical conditions of management, housing, nutrition and season of the year. This is impossible to achieve and so a variation in results, even between different flocks on the same farm, often occurs. Turkeys do not lay as well in hot weather as in cold weather. Any breeder's specification therefore can only be an assessment of average field results and as such can only be used as a guide. It is not uncommon for flock farmers to regularly exceed the specifications. Others do not achieve them. During any investigation it is important to check with each company how they arrive at their records of production. Egg production may be recorded as total eggs laid or as settable eggs, which will exclude cracked or misshapen eggs, those with poor shell quality and eggs weighing below 65 g. Hatchability may be recorded as all poults obtained, including 'help outs', or as numbers of first-class poults.

Egg collection should occur at least five times daily, including a late afternoon collection. Floor eggs should be collected and kept separate and if set, set separately. Immediate sanitation of all hatching eggs by either fumigation or washing using a special machine is done on many farms. Emphasis, however, should be on production of clean eggs not on sanitization as bacteria penetrate the shell before this can be effected.

Storage of eggs should be within the range 13–18 °C (55–65 °F) with relative humidity of 65–70%.

When set the egg should be less than 8 days old. Thereafter the hatchability reduces fairly quickly. Storage in plastic bags and inert gases reduces this deterioration considerably.

Turkey eggs vary in colour. Some flocks lay many white and/or misshapen eggs that do not hatch as well as the others. This may be due to stress, physical upsets, parasitism or disease.

Mortality during the fattening period is very variable within the industry: 3.5–12% without any specific diseases are the extremes. It should be less than 1% in the first week.

For breeding flocks it is estimated that for every 1000 birds required for laying, 1200 day-old poults are purchased. In other words it is expected that the number of day-old poults will be reduced due to culling of unsuitable birds and mortality. Many people achieve better results than this. The figure is much higher for stags, which are put under much greater selection pressures. Two hundred and fifty day-olds are bought for every 100 adult stags required.

During lay hen mortality is normally very low (0.1% per week), slightly more as the flock is coming into production, mainly due to prolapse and yolk peritonitis.

Disease prevention

Vaccination

Birds may be vaccinated twice with live Newcastle disease (ND) vaccine in the water or by aerosol at 4 and 7 weeks of age. Breeding flocks also receive inactivated oil emulsion ND vaccine at 10 weeks and again at 28 weeks. Breeders are sometimes vaccinated against fowl pox on the insides of the thigh, not in the wing web. They sleep with their heads under the wings and develop lesions on their face if vaccination is done in the wing web.

Some breeders are also vaccinated against paramyxovirus 3 (PMV3) infection, twice at an interval of 4 weeks, the last being given 2 weeks before the flock comes into lay.

Live turkey rhinotracheitis vaccine is given to young poults from 5 days of age by aerosol or eye drop. Birds must be kept in good environmental conditions and must not be debeaked within 10 days following the vaccination. An inactivated vaccine may be developed for the breeders. Problem farms may require birds to be vaccinated against erysipelas and/or pasteurellosis. There is a combined vaccine that must be administered twice, with an interval of 3–4 weeks between doses, the last one being given approximately 2 weeks before expected problems and the first not earlier than 6 weeks of age. In the case of breeders it is repeated a third time just before point of lay. The efficiency of pasteurella vaccination is not very good due to the multiplicity of strains not covered by the vaccines.

Coccidiostats

Coccidiostats, for example monensin, lasalocid, halofuginone, amprolium and amprolium/sulphaquinoxaline mixtures, are administered in feed usually until 8 weeks of age but recent work has indicated that under some conditions it is worthwhile continuing until 12 weeks of age with fattening birds. The ionophores, except lasalocid, are highly toxic to adult turkeys and should be used in fattening stock with care. Tiamulin and chloramphenicol can increase the toxicity of these drugs.

Anti-blackhead (histomoniasis) drugs are often given in the feed throughout the life of the birds. However, on many farms blackhead is no longer a problem since the advent of concrete floored, controlled-environment houses, and anti-blackhead drugs are not given. In some operations anti-blackhead drug is fed from 2 to 6 weeks of age to control a 'necrotic enteritis' type condition. Farms that produce the best results are all-in/all-out one-age farms. Some sites have 300 000 birds on them. Multi-age farms have, inevitably, more problems.

As with all intensive livestock keeping, isolation of sites, site security, hygiene, interbatch clean out and disinfection are of paramount importance in reducing disease risks and in improving performance. One cannot rely on vaccination or medication alone.

General management

Management decisions made by the owner and their implementation by the stockperson will be reflected in the health of any turkey flock. This is especially so when birds are housed intensively and are entirely dependent on man for the necessities of life, i.e. feed, water, warmth, fresh air and protection from uncontrolled disease. Any effect on the health of the turkey flock should always be considered when looking at the geographical siting, house design, construction, purchase of day-old stock and day-to-day procedures. Individuals within each flock have slightly different requirements and abilities to respond to the environment. Many problems of poor production and/or mortality arise because these basic facts are not fully appreciated. The probability of the flock becoming unhealthy as well as its ability to recover or not, are greatly influenced by such management considerations.

Disease, as an impairment to normal body functions, may occur due to infection or infestation with agents such as bacteria, viruses, mycoplasmas, fungi or parasites, or as a result of nutritional deficiencies, toxic substances, injuries or stress. From time to time new conditions arise of unknown aetiology. Where infectious or parasitic agents are involved the severity of the disease will depend upon the complex interaction between the host bird, the infectious agent and the general management. In other cases the severity of disease is determined by the extent of nutritional deficiency, the amount of toxic substances ingested or the extent of any injury. Good management may alleviate the effect of these conditions but inadequate management will precipitate and aggravate them.

It is vitally important where disease, increased mortality and reduced production occur that help is sought quickly by the farmer in order that a competent diagnosis is made and steps taken to alleviate the situation as soon as possible. Experienced personnel may recognize many conditions from the signs and post-mortem pictures; however, many conditions require more sophisticated laboratory investigations before a precise diagnosis can be made and confirmed. The help of a veterinary diagnostic laboratory should therefore be sought as soon as possible.

Any poultry keeper who understands and carries out the basic management practices that prevent outbreaks of disease has little need to know the detailed knowledge of signs, lesions and medications for individual diseases.

Where large concentrations of birds and high capital commitment are involved monitoring of vaccination programmes by serological tests, and monitoring of litter, feed samples and general hygiene are all important. However, monitoring for monitoring's sake is a waste of time and effort. The results must be constantly reviewed, assessed as a whole and changes made to specific procedures if the results are not as would be expected.

It is estimated that at least 50% of problems, especially in young birds, are related to management faults rather than disease outbreaks.

Therapeutic medication may be necessary once a diagnosis has been obtained if the cause is due to a bacterium. Antibiotic sensitivity tests are useful in indicating which antibacterial drug may be effective. However, they are not foolproof. There may be overlying management faults such as inadequate ventilation, overstocking or viral infections such as turkey rhinotracheitis, which tend to nullify the effect of any antibacterial therapy.

It should be remembered that sick birds tend to drink rather than eat so initial medication should always be via the drinking water. This can usually be applied much more quickly than via the feed, which requires special mixing and inevitable delays. However, if extended treatment is required, medication by the feed after the initial water medication is preferable.

Whichever method of medication is used, full therapeutic doses for the recommended period should be given. Reduced dosage rates for short periods can lead to the development of resistant organisms, which can perpetuate the disease outbreak and make further outbreaks more difficult to control. Under present UK legislation, in-feed anti-bacterial medications may only be supplied with a Veterinary Written Direction issued by the veterinary surgeon who has recently visited the site and performed post-mortems on some of the birds.

When selecting the drug it is necessary to remember that many are not absorbed from the intestine and that these must only be used for treating intestinal problems, e.g. neomycin and penicillin. The absorption of some others, such as oxytetracycline and chlortetracycline, is somewhat impaired by high calcium levels in the feed.

Drugs are rarely administered by injection although it may be necessary in cases of erysipelas and fowl cholera to inject some flocks.

Therapeutic treatment, if effective, produces a fairly rapid response. If there is no improvement within five days it is unlikely that any response will be forthcoming. In this case the diagnosis, treatment, dosage rate and method of administration must be reassessed.

Important diseases of turkeys

Aortic rupture (dissecting aneurysm)

The cause of this is not fully established though implantation with stilboestrol, toxic factors in certain seeds, genetic factors and the normally high blood pressure in turkeys combined with stress, high levels of protein and fat in the diet and/or the endotoxin of *Candida albicans* have all been suggested as possible causes.

Sudden death in birds over 10 weeks of age could be caused by this condition. Usually the percentage in the flock that dies is fairly small but on occasions it can be as high as 2%. The major artery of the body, the aorta, ruptures near the gonads causing sudden death that may occasionally be preceded by gasping or blood running from the mouth. The head, skin and muscles appear pale. The abdominal cavity is filled with large blood clots.

Occasionally the renal arteries rupture and there is a massive blood clot under the kidney capsule. In this case the birds are not pale and death is more likely due to shock.

There is no specific treatment. The use of tranquillizers such as reserpine has been tried with varying success. Reducing the level of protein and feeding up to 120 ppm of copper as copper sulphate is also said to help.

Arizona infection

This infection is caused by a motile bacterium, *Arizona hinshawii* (formerly called *Salmonella arizonae*). It bears a very close relationship to the *Salmonella* genus. The aetiology and epidemiology are very similar to that of the salmonella group. Both vertical and lateral transmission occur. Vermin, feed and house and hatchery environments can all be sources of contamination. Adults and birds over five weeks of age rarely show any signs. Those below five weeks may look very ill with diarrhoea and some will be blind, show nervous signs and possibly paralysis. Mortality varies between 10% and 50%. Many of the survivors are stunted and unthrifty. On post-mortem one finds the generalized septicaemic lesions of serofibrinous pericarditis and perihepatitis with occasional caecal plugs and caseous exudates in the abdominal cavity and a whitish-yellow pus in the posterior chamber of the eye. Bacteriological examination in the laboratory is necessary to distinguish this organism from salmonellae. In the adult, one may have to resort to serological tests to determine whether the flock is infected or not.

Treatment is with antibiotics, including furazolidone (with or without neomycin), tetracycline, quinolones and sulphonamides; results are extremely variable. The injection of day-old poults in enzootic areas is usually carried out but again with variable results; gentamycin, spectinomycin, tetracyclines or a combination of streptomycin and penicillin are all being used for injecting day-old poults.

Arizona infection is not found in the UK. Any flocks that in the past were contaminated have been slaughtered. However, the possibility of this disease should always be considered where young blind poults are seen amongst sick birds showing nervous signs. It should not be confused with *Salmonella typhimurium* or *Salmonella enteriditis*.

Ascaridia infection (large roundworms, *Ascaris*, ascariasis)

Ascaridia dissimilis is a species of large, white tapered roundworms with one end curled, that are found free within the intestinal tract. The adults lay eggs that are passed in the droppings. After 10–14 days, in warm and moist conditions, larvae develop within the egg which is then infective if ingested by a bird. These larvae may remain viable for 4 or 5 years if they are not eaten. Once the egg has been eaten the larva breaks out and penetrates the wall of the intestine, where it remains for a few days before entering the intestinal lumen to live on the digesta. The parasites may affect the bird by removing nutrients or by massive larval infiltration of the intestinal tract or by blocking the intestinal tract due to the presence of large numbers of adult worms. It takes approximately 50 days for the newly ingested infective larva to develop into an adult worm capable of laying an egg.

Small numbers of these worms are not important but heavy infestations may retard the growth of fattening birds and lower production in layer flocks. The latter often lay white-shelled eggs.

Treatment with piperazine is very effective and safe. The calculated amount of drug should be given for a few hours in the drinking water after a short period of water deprivation. Piperazine narcotizes the adult worms, which pass out in the faeces and die outside the host. They are not infective to birds. Only adult worms are affected, so it is necessary to repeat the treatment at three-weekly intervals to eliminate immature forms which have become adults.

Levamisole and mebendazole are effective against both mature and immature stages of the parasite.

The eggs of these worms are extremely resistant and persistent. It is almost impossible to remove them from earth floors but with concrete floors the use of 5% ammonia during the cleanout will help to control them. However, the infective worm eggs can easily be carried on footwear back into a house from contaminated surrounds.

Aspergillosis (brooder pneumonia)

This is caused by the mould *Aspergillus fumigatus*, which produces large numbers of very resistant spores; these can be found in the air in virtually any farming operation. Occasionally *A. glaucus* and *A. niger* are involved. There are more problems with aspergillosis after a poor harvest as the source of infection is frequently mouldy hay, straw or other organic matter or the feed. Clinical disease only occurs when birds inhale large numbers of spores over a short period of time. This could happen when there is gross contamination of the environment of the hatchery or rearing house, or of the litter or feed. The spores gain entry via cracks in the shell to the inside of a hatching egg where they multiply in the air cell and kill off the embryo. If the egg is broken large numbers of spores are released into the atmosphere. Extremely heavy losses in poults may occur during the first week of life when this occurs.

The young poult is most severely affected during the first few days after hatching. However, the spores do not pass from bird to bird so mortality usually ceases between 10 and 12 days of age. The birds will be found to be gasping, usually without making any sounds, about 5 days after exposure. All such infected poults die within a couple of weeks. Occasionally, a few weeks later nervous signs may be seen in a few survivors—ataxia, falling or pushing themselves over backwards, paralysis and bending the head over the back. On rare occasions there may be a caseous pellet under the nictitatory membrane where birds are showing an ocular discharge. Older birds of any age may cough, become weak and show difficulty in breathing, especially if disturbed, and will eventually die.

In young birds there is a collection of small yellowish nodules in the lungs and air sacs. These nodules tend to be grey and granuloma-like in the lungs of older birds. In the air sacs concave button-shaped plaques are often seen with greeny blue-black centres. Nervous signs are accompanied by yellowish-white fairly large lesions in the brain. The fungus can be readily isolated from any of these lesions.

There is no treatment other than to remove the source of contamination.

Avian influenza

Many different serological types of the influenza A group have been identified as causing problems in turkeys, resulting in a very variable clinical picture. Outbreaks tend to occur often without the source of infection being discovered. Wild birds, especially ducks and imported exotics, are thought to act as reservoirs.

The very virulent members of this group cause the condition known as fowl plague and may cause up to 100% mortality. It is suspected that humans, horses and pigs may become infected by some strains of avian influenza A virus.

The signs of the infection are extremely variable. Usually the flock becomes lethargic, goes very quiet and is off its feed for two or three days. There may be nervous signs with the birds becoming paralysed and often dying in convulsions. Respiratory signs may be very mild or very severe, with coughing, sneezing, conjunctivitis, sinusitis and swelling of the head and the face. A moderate to severe temporary drop in egg production occurs and a number of chalky unpigmented or soft-shelled eggs may be laid. Fertility and hatchability are sometimes depressed. Mortality may occur over a period of 5–6 days. In adults it is often due to an egg peritonitis. Mortality will vary from virtually nothing to as much as 70% but is usually in the lower region. Spread through the farm is usually fairly slow but related to the movement of personnel. Sudden changes in weather or concurrent disease such as mycoplasmosis will increase the severity of the disease. Recovered flocks show a serological response.

The lesions found in affected birds vary with the clinical signs observed. They are mainly restricted to the respiratory tract with congested lungs, air sacculitis and sinusitis.

The history and the signs may be suggestive of this infection but virological and serological procedures are necessary to confirm the diagnosis. Cloacal swabs are a useful source of the virus. The different serotypes of the influenza A virus can rapidly undergo recombination and mutation.

Flocks free from *Mycoplasma gallisepticum* sometimes show a transient non-specific reaction to the rapid plate test for *M. gallisepticum* when challenged with an influenza A virus as well as showing a sinusitis.

Treatment is not specific but aimed at the secondary infections and removal of stress factors.

In most countries there is no effective vaccine because there are so many different serotypes of the virus. Some countries do permit the use of an autogenous inactivated vaccine. It is essential to prevent contact between wild birds and flocks of turkeys. Nonetheless, outbreaks do occur in controlled-environment houses. There has been no evidence of egg transmission.

Fowl plague is a notifiable disease in most countries, and infected flocks are compulsorily slaughtered.

Blepharo conjunctivitis

The cause of this condition is not known but it is suspected that it may be dust entering the eyes, especially of birds coming into lay, which causes a white frothy foam in the inner canthus of the eyes. Secondary bacterial infections follow. The birds rub their eyes along the feathers over their shoulders causing further irritation. These events, together with pecking by the other birds, result in severe damage to the eyelids often leading to complete destruction of the eyeball itself. The eyelids become thickened and distorted by scar tissue. There is no direct treatment but infected birds should be removed at once otherwise the pecking of the eyes becomes a habit and a vice within the flock. Daily treatment with an ophthalmic ointment usually aids recovery.

Coccidiosis

Nine species of *Eimeria* are found in turkeys, none of which affect chickens, although the coccidia of the two hosts show similar life cycles. Four are thought to be capable of causing disease, and two are very pathogenic, *E. adenoides* and *E. meleagrimitis*. It is rare to see any clinical problems after eight weeks of age although oocysts are frequently found in the faeces of older turkeys that may show impaired growth or suboptimal feed conversion.

The birds appear dejected, tend to huddle in groups near the source of heat and stop eating. Only a few birds or a large proportion of the flock may be affected. Mortality may be high or there may only be impaired growth rate.

Post-mortem findings show a swollen duodenum with gelatinous contents where *E. meleagrimitis* is involved. The caeca may contain white cheesy cores, consisting of masses of oocysts in cases of *E. adenoides* infestation.

Other conditions may be mistaken for coccidiosis and therefore a competent laboratory diagnosis is essential. If only a few oocysts are present it is unlikely that coccidiosis is causing the problem. Only where massive numbers of oocysts occur can it be assumed that the condition is purely due to coccidiosis. Coccidiosis must be distinguished from necrotic enteritis caused by *Clostridium perfringens*, where the contents of the intestine may be full of necrotic material.

Treatment with potentiated sulphonamide drugs or one of the amprolium drugs is usually effective. All are administered in drinking water and must be given as directed by the manufacturer's instructions. Turkeys have very definite likes and dislikes and will refuse to drink if any of the drugs are given at even slightly above the recommended dose rate.

If the condition does not clear up it is possible that necrotic enteritis is also present and the diagnosis must be reassessed.

Where outbreaks of coccidiosis have occurred it is advisable to include a washdown with a 10% solution of commercially available ammonia solution at the end of interbatch cleanout and disinfection. This should involve all possible sources of contamination, including floors, walls, feedstores and protective clothing and footwear.

During the life of the flock damp patches in the litter must be avoided and so must anything that causes a reduction in the feed intake. An anticoccidial drug should be included in the feed for at least eight weeks although there are indications that benefits may be derived by extending this to 12 weeks in some circumstances.

As with other species of animals the specific coccidia do become resistant to drugs so the anticoccidial drug has to be periodically changed. Several are available but availability will vary from country to country. The three most widely used in the UK are: Elancoban (Elanco Products Ltd; monensin); Stenerol (Hoechst UK Ltd; halofuginone); and Avatec (Roche Ltd; lasalocid).

Egg peritonitis (yolk peritonitis)

This occurs where the ovulating follicle is deposited free in the abdominal cavity instead of into the infundibulum of the oviduct. In many cases the yolk is resorbed and nothing further occurs. In other cases the yolk is broken and peritonitis develops.

The risk of yolk peritonitis may be increased by:

1. Physical damage due to mishandling of the birds.
2. Respiratory infections, especially where primary exposure to *Mycoplasma gallisepticum* or avian influenza is involved.

3. Stress of the birds as they come naturally into lay.
4. Ascending infections of the oviduct.

Birds usually die in fairly good condition after a few days of illness. Occasionally some develop chronic lesions and gradually lose condition until they are culled or die.

In acute cases the birds are usually dehydrated showing very dark musculature and reduced pliability of the skin. There will be a whitish-yellow cheesy exudate surrounding the organs of the abdominal cavity, many of which are stuck together with adhesions.

There is no specific treatment available but it is necessary to identify and remove any predisposing cause. Antibiotic treatment may reduce the number of acute deaths but usually increases the number of chronic cases.

Erysipelas

This is an acute bacterial disease caused by *Erysipelothrix insidiosa*. This organism is widely distributed and found in many animals, including turkeys, ducks, chickens, water fowl, wild birds, pigs, sheep, rodents and fish. Turkeys and pigs are the most susceptible. It can cause a cellulitis and skin rash in humans.

E. insidiosa can survive for long periods in the soil. Damage to the skin by biting insects, fighting, pecking or cannibalism will introduce infection into the individual bird, and artificial insemination techniques have also been incriminated. Sometimes a sudden change to cold wet weather has also been associated with an outbreak. Contaminated fish meal has been known to introduce infection onto farms.

Erysipelas is mainly a disease of older heavier birds and is rarely seen before 13 weeks of age. It is often restricted to one pen in the house, spreading slowly to the others. Mortality can vary from under 1% to 50%.

The condition is usually acute, causing death in birds in good condition with very little or no prior illness. Frequently the owners suspect poisoning. Laying hens may be found dead on the nest. If a bird is seen before it dies it looks lethargic and has an unsteady gait. On rare occasions chronic cases develop that show scabby necrotic skin lesions especially on the snood, which may also be swollen and purplish in colour.

In acute cases small haemorrhages may be found in the skin, muscles, pericardial fat, gizzard serosa, mesentery and under the pleura. Frequently a catarrhal enteritis is present. The liver and spleen are usually enlarged and friable and the kidneys are swollen. In peracute cases no lesions may be found. Occasionally in chronic cases, especially if birds have been vaccinated, small yellowish cauliflower-like growths may be found on the lining or valves of the heart.

Bacterial laboratory examinations are required to confirm the presence of this disease.

A specific treatment is available. The birds in the group showing mortality should be injected with a mixture of procaine penicillin (rapid-acting) and benzathine penicillin (long-acting). From a different syringe, but at the same time, they should also be given a dose of erysipelas vaccine. The injections should be given subcutaneously at the base of the neck to avoid abscesses or blemishes in the musculature. Remaining members of the flock not showing any mortality need only be given the vaccine, which in all cases must be repeated after 3–4 weeks. If the flock is to be slaughtered within 10–14 days of the penicillin treatment there is no need to vaccinate.

It is essential when injecting the birds that the needle used for birds in the pen in which there is mortality is not used for those which are not infected. Medication via the feed or water is usually ineffective in acute cases. Turkeys should not be reared close to pigs or in buildings or on land which have previously been used for pigs or sheep.

Where *Erysipelothrix* infection is enzootic the turkeys will need to be vaccinated with the inactivated vaccine, which is often combined with one for *Pasteurella multocida*.

The vaccine is administered subcutaneously at the back of the neck or intramuscularly in the breast muscle. A repeat dose is necessary three to four weeks later. The turkeys can be vaccinated at any age from six weeks onwards; however, it is necessary to ensure that the vaccination is timed so that the second dose is given two weeks before outbreaks of erysipelas usually occur. This ensures that each bird has its highest level of immunity when it is most needed.

Erysipelas vaccine occasionally stimulates non-specific serum plate agglutination reactions to *Mycoplasma gallisepticum* and *M. meleagridis*, which may persist for several days. It is not advisable to take routine monitoring serum samples for these conditions within a fortnight of the birds being vaccinated for erysipelas.

E. coli infections (colibacillosis, coliform infection)

Escherichia coli are normal inhabitants of the intestinal tract in all animals and birds and hence are present in large numbers in the environment, dust and litter of the poultry house. There are many different serotypes but usually only three (01, 02 and 078) are true pathogens and cause primary disease. Other serotypes are opportunists which cause problems as secondary invaders following either viral infections or stress due to management problems. Often, secondary colibacillosis is more harmful to the bird than a primary virus infection, as in the case of rhinotracheitis.

The *E. coli* bacteria penetrate the tissues of the respiratory and intestinal tracts damaged by infections or irritations and thus invade the bloodstream to cause an *E. coli* bacteraemia. Thus *E. coli* bacteraemia is associated with respiratory conditions due to Newcastle disease, avian influenza, turkey rhinotracheitis and mycoplasmosis as well as with management factors such as overcrowding, under-ventilating, chilling and very dry, dusty atmospheres.

As with all bacterial diseases the birds may die very quickly or they may be ill for a few days, standing around hunched and looking very miserable, often huddling towards any heat source, or hiding under drinkers or feeders, or along the walls of the house. Birds usually die on their breasts, often trampled on by other birds.

Typical septicaemic lesions are found in young birds, with whitish-yellow serofibrinous deposits on the pericardium, around the liver and in the air sacs. In older birds the liver and spleen are usually swollen and congested and rapidly change to a dark greenish colour on exposure to the air. Small haemorrhages may be seen in the liver, under the gizzard serosa and occasionally in the heart fat in acute cases. Others will show a serofibrinous air sacculitis and pericarditis especially if *Mycoplasma gallisepticum* is also present. A serofibrinous perihepatitis is uncommon in older turkeys.

E. coli may also be involved in tumour-like masses known as coligranulomata that occur along the intestinal tract and in the liver, in yolk sac infections and in cases of salpingitis, synovitis, arthritis, breast blisters, enteritis and peritonitis.

Antibacterial therapy can be useful, preferably with a drug given in the drinking water, where a sensitivity test has shown the organism to be sensitive to that drug. This therapy is unlikely to be effective if the primary cause is not also corrected.

Haemorrhagic enteritis

A member of the adenovirus family has been implicated by many workers as the causal agent of this condition. It is very widespread in turkeys and most flocks in the UK convert serologically between 8 and 12 weeks of age. Mortality may be quite high but is usually fairly low. Young turkeys under four weeks of age appear resistant to the disease.

Outbreaks may be precipitated by overcrowding, chilling or inadequate nutrition. In these cases the birds may go off their legs sitting 'doglike' on their hocks and show dark tarry droppings. In more acute cases there is sudden death in flocks of 8–14 weeks of age over a period of 5–10 days. Occasionally bloody droppings are seen soiling the vent feathers. These birds at post-mortem show massive haemorrhaging into the intestines, starting in the duodenum but frequently extending along the whole length of the intestine. Survivors have enlarged mottled spleens that persist for various lengths of time; these are frequently seen on the processing line. Susceptible breeding stock challenged with this virus will show a drop in egg production and an increased incidence of white thin-shelled eggs.

Histological examination of the spleen, intestine and other organs will reveal small intranuclear inclusion bodies in the reticuloendothelial cells. An agar gel precipitation test may be used to detect the virus or antibodies to the virus.

There is no specific treatment although serum prepared from recovered clinical cases administered by injection affords considerable protection.

Vaccines are available in some countries such as France, but not in the UK. Management practices must ensure that the birds are of adequate nutritional status and are not subjected to stresses of chilling or overcrowding.

There is a good deal of evidence that the causal agent is the same virus that causes marble spleen disease in pheasants.

Hepatosis (ascites)

This occurs in birds of between 10 and 30 days of age. The causes are unknown although coal tar disinfectants, aflatoxin, furazolidone, poisoning with nitrosamines, chlorinated hydrocarbons or wood preservatives in the litter, and stress factors such as chilling and overheating have been implicated. It should not be confused with salt poisoning, toxic fat syndrome or exudative diathesis (vitamin E/selenium deficiency), which show similar but distinguishable post-mortem lesions.

Mortality may be up to 25% of the flock. Those that die are usually good birds that are showing drowsiness and disinclination to move for 1–2 days before dying. Some will show respiratory distress but do not make any respiratory noises. The majority of the flock progresses fairly normally.

The abdomens are swollen with large amounts of watery fluid, which is also present in the lungs, pericardial sac, musculature and in severe cases under the skin. The heart is frequently enlarged. The liver is usually relatively small and hard and may be rounded and congested.

Often when this condition has occurred in the flock there is another increase in mortality at 4–6 weeks of age, when well-grown birds die showing ascites, cirrhotic livers and very enlarged thin-walled round hearts.

There is no effective treatment.

Heterakis infestation (caecal worms)

Heterakis gallinarum is a small threadlike roundworm, 1–2 cm (½–¾ in) long, commonly found in the caecae of turkeys. It has a similar life cycle to the ascarids: under favourable conditions the larvae break out of the eggs when these are eaten by the host and develop into adult worms in the caeca. The eggs may remain viable in earthworms and soil for a long period.

The worms are found mostly in turkeys kept on earth floors. They themselves are of little importance but they act as a means of transmission of the histomonad parasite that causes histomoniasis (blackhead) (see below).

Levamisole and mebendazole are effective against both mature and larval stages. Phenothiazine is only effective against the adult worms.

Histomoniasis (blackhead, enterohepatitis)

This is caused by the parasite *Histomonas meleagridis*, a flagellated protozoan that survives only for a few hours outside the body of the hosts—turkey, peafowl, chickens, pheasants and guinea fowl. However, it may be transmitted encased within the eggs of the parasitic roundworm *Heterakis gallinarum* in such a form that it may survive in the soil or in earthworms for many years. Secondary bacteria infection helps to create the caecal lesions seen in this condition.

Histomoniasis in young poults is an acute, fatal, rapidly spreading disease. In older birds it is less acute, spreading more slowly, and in some cases may be relatively chronic. Typically, affected birds are drowsy, with dropped wings and often soiled vent feathers due to a sulphur-yellow coloured diarrhoea. These signs occur 15–21 days after exposure. Cyanosis of the head (blackhead) is rarely seen.

The initial lesion in the caecae is a severe inflammation, sometimes haemorrhagic, with thickened walls that are distended with gelatinous to solid caecal cores which show concentric rings when cut. Ulcers may form, some of which may penetrate the wall of the caeca to create a peritonitis that frequently produces a second upsurge in mortality after supposedly successful treatment. Caecal lesions may be the only ones seen in acute cases. The secondary liver lesions consist of circular depressed areas of necrotic tissue that are greyish-yellow in colour. In the young poult these may be diffuse and whitish in colour. Demonstration of the infective parasite can be quite difficult.

Treatment with dimetridazole in the drinking water followed by the same or another anti-blackhead drug in the feed is very effective. However, no immunity to histomoniasis develops so the anti-blackhead drug must be fed until slaughter.

Where histomoniasis is a problem the turkeys should be given an anti-histomonad drug in the feed from three weeks until slaughter. The introduction of concrete floors in controlled-environment houses has reduced the need for preventive medication on many farms.

Occasionally there are breakdowns even when the birds are on medicated feed. This usually occurs because there has been inadequate mixing of the drug or some factor such as disease or a management fault has reduced the feed intake of the birds, for instance when the diet is supplemented by grain, straw or grass. The marked increase in the number of earthworms rising to the soil surface after heavy rainfall may produce a very heavy parasite challenge and cause problems in free-range turkeys.

Lymphoproliferative disease (LPD)

This may cause high mortality in up to 20% of birds from seven weeks onwards. Different strains of turkeys vary in their response to this challenge. Frequently the onset of mortality is associated with stress factors such as moving, concurrent disease or high stocking densities. Males are affected more than females. Sporadic cases appear in adult breeders. The exact cause or mode of transmission of the disease are uncertain but vertical transmission may play a part since it frequently occurs in successive batches of poults on all-in/all-out sites. Even though the causal agent has not been isolated inoculation of spleen from clinical cases produces the clinical disease. Strong circumstantial evidence suggests that this is caused by a type c virus of the family Retroviridae.

Some of the birds are ill, standing about and not eating, for a few days before they die. Even so the birds are usually in good condition. The characteristic lesion is an extremely enlarged whitish spleen, variously described as marbled or salami sausage-like. Sometimes the liver is slightly enlarged with small white foci scattered throughout the organ. Similar but small lesions may be found in the lungs, proventriculus, pancreas, testes, ovary and thymus. On rare occasions enlarged peripheral nerves are found. The incidence of aortic rupture is frequently higher in LPD-affected flocks than in non-affected flocks.

There is no known treatment other than avoiding stress factors, having good standards of hygiene and avoiding susceptible strains of birds.

Lice and mite infestation

Lice are rarely a problem unless present in very large numbers, when they may depress egg production and cause irritation to the flock attendants and to the AI team. They spend their entire life cycle on the bird, feeding on skin and feather debris.

Mite infestation, like that of lice, is not as common as formerly.

Red Mite (Dermanyssus gallinae)

These small mites attack the birds at night and are vicious bloodsuckers.

During the day they hide in cracks and crevices of the buildings, making it difficult to find them on the birds. Blood-stained eggs are usually the first sign that they may be present.

Northern Fowl Mite (Ornithonyssus sylvarum)

This small mite stays on the bird. It is also a vicious bloodsucker, attacking mainly the vent area, which becomes reddened and may show darkened scabs. It is a more common parasite in turkeys than the red mite. Blood loss with both these parasites will affect production.

Control measures

Lice and mites are effectively controlled by insecticides such as sevin and malathion. There are also many other preparations on the market. Dusting the breeding stock at the time of AI is effective. Since the red mite hides in cracks and crevices, the walls and nest boxes must also be treated with the insecticide. It is important that treatments are repeated after two weeks and thereafter monthly as they are only effective against the adult mite, not against eggs or larval stages. It is also important that the manufacturer's recommendations are closely followed otherwise toxic effects may occur. After heavy infestations the application of creosote to nest boxes, walls and roof supports greatly reduces any carryover to the next flock.

Muscle myopathy (Oregon Muscle Disease, Green Muscle Disease, Deep Pectoral Myopathy, Degenerative Myopathy of Turkeys)

This is primarily a condition in which muscle tissue dies due to failure in its blood supply. No infective agent is involved. It is mainly seen in end-of-production breeders but is becoming more and more common in large fattening birds. The deep pectoral muscle (deep fillet) is trapped between an inelastic fascia and the bony sternum thus preventing the normal physiological swelling that occurs when muscles are exercised. This leads to strangulation of the blood vessels within the muscle and the resulting lesion.

The lesions are usually only seen on the processing line and may be unilateral or bilateral. They are rarely detected in the live bird. In advanced cases the breast appears flattened rather than the normal rounded shape. This specific lesion occurs around a band of fascia that runs through the deep pectoral muscle. The area affected is variable in size. Initially there is a swollen reddish brown lesion which later becomes green and shrunken and then pale green. It is possible to find the lesion by palpation but a cold light source must be inserted into the body cavity of the carcase in a darkened room to be sure of detecting all lesions. This is frequently done in end-of-lay flocks.

No public health significance is attached to the lesion but it is aesthetically undesirable. The fillet should be removed but the rest of the carcase is fit for human consumption, usually as a further processed product.

Mycoplasmosis

Four species of the genus *Mycoplasma* cause problems with turkeys: *M. gallisepticum*, *M. meleagridis*, *M. synoviae* and *M. iowae*. The major breeds are now free of *M. gallisepticum*. Eradication has been obtained by rearing small groups in isolation aided by medicinal treatment of the breeding stock, hatching eggs and day-old poults. The whole operation has to be rigorously controlled by serological monitoring of the progeny for freedom from the infection.

The other species are gradually being eradicated but unfortunately at the moment there is no serological test for *M. iowae*.

Mycoplasmas are very delicate organisms that are easily killed outside the host. Spread is mainly vertical through eggs laid by carrier birds followed by some lateral spread between birds kept in close contact or on heavily populated sites. *M. meleagridis* is also spread venereally.

Hatching eggs from infected parents are usually subjected to immersion in tylosin solution under vacuum in an attempt to reduce egg transmission.

Mycoplasma gallisepticum *infection (Infectious Sinusitis)*

This organism is involved with the chronic respiratory disease (CRD) complex of chickens, turkeys, game birds and pigeons. It may lie dormant in birds causing no problems until triggered off by some stress factor or other disease.

M. gallisepticum will increase the severity of any reaction to Newcastle disease live virus vaccines and other respiratory signs, especially those due to poor environmental conditions, resulting in reduced growth rates and downgrading of carcases. Affected birds cough and sneeze and show swellings of one or both infraorbital sinuses and may show a cloudy viscous exudate from the nostrils. Frequently feathers covering the back and the base of the wings are soiled because the birds rub the swollen sinuses over their backs. These swellings may be so large that they close the eyes. Severely affected birds lose weight whilst others show a reduced weight gain, depending on environmental factors. Adult flocks that become affected by mycoplasmosis while in lay may show reduced egg production and increased yolk peritonitis.

The swollen sinuses are full of greyish viscous fluid which later becomes caseous. There is a varying degree of air sacculitis, ranging from cloudy air sacs to a seropurulent exudate. Usually clinical signs bear little relationship to the degree of air sacculitis. Frequently, secondary *E. coli* infections occur which complicate the condition and lead to a generalized *E. coli* septicaemia with a serofibrinous perihepatitis, pericarditis, pneumonia and increased mortality.

Young turkey poults may show abnormal bone formation, retarded growth, abnormal feather development and reduced liveability if they are infected via the egg.

M. gallisepticum infection should be suspected where respiratory signs are associated with swollen sinuses. Confirmation can be done by isolation of the agent and paired serological tests. However, false positives may occur in serological tests so an awareness of the vagaries of interpretations is necessary.

Swollen sinuses may also occur unrelated to *M. gallisepticum* infection in dusty atmospheres and during outbreaks of influenza A infection.

Treatment with antibiotics and the macrolide drugs are useful though they may not be economically worth while unless mortality is occurring or there is severe weight loss. Treatment will need to be repeated. In severe cases it is frequently also necessary to include medication for secondary *E. coli* infection.

Mycoplasma synoviae *infection (Infectious Synovitis)*

This usually causes fewer flock problems in turkeys unless a very virulent strain is present. The same stress factors as highlighted with *M. gallisepticum* also precipitate clinical symptoms with *M. synoviae*. Clinical signs include depression, poor growth and lameness due to swellings in the hock and foot joints and occasionally in the tendons. Breast blisters are common in turkeys and are frequently, though not invariably, associated with *M. synoviae* infection. Diagnosis once again is by the use of serological tests or by isolating the organisms.

Severely affected birds should be culled. The remainder of the flock may be treated with high levels of chlortetracycline or the macrolide drugs.

Mycoplasma meleagridis *infection*

This organism is widespread in turkey flocks and may be present on the phallus and in the oviduct of mature birds, or in the cloaca and bursa of Fabricius in younger birds without necessarily causing any damage to the organs. Spread is via the egg and venereally, which highlights the special care needed during artificial insemination. Infection reduces hatchability, and causes twisted necks and abnormalities in bone and feather growth. Air sacculitis is also seen in young poults, which reduces liveability. This infection, especially if aggravated by high brooding temperatures, has led to a condition known as 'TS 65'. The birds are stunted but usually have good muscular development, with or without bowing of the legs, and many broken brittle feathers. Affected birds should be culled.

Once again diagnosis is usually based on clinical signs, isolation of the organism and serological tests.

Treatment is not very effective once the clinical signs have appeared.

Mycoplasma iowae

This organism has been shown to produce lowered hatchability when injected into embryos, and depressed growth. It is very widespread in turkeys but its significance is not fully understood in the field. Breeding organizations are trying to eliminate it from the stock. Repeated treatments of breeding flocks with Baytril (enrofloxacin) is said to increase the number of viable poults produced.

Necrotic enteritis

This is a condition in which large numbers of *Clostridium perfringens* bacteria multiply in the intestines and cause swelling of the intestinal wall, ulceration, and necrosis of the mucosal cells resulting in pinky-brown necrotic debris in the lumen.

A few coccidial oocysts may be demonstrated in intestinal smears in the affected area. Although these may be the initial trigger factor, the condition responds better to oral administration of dimetridazole, penicillin or erythromycin rather than anticoccidial drugs.

The condition tends to recur in successive flocks over the period of 3–6 weeks of age. Problem sites usually administer dimetridazole in the feed over this susceptible period. Hygiene precautions during interbatch cleanout should be vigorously enforced to reduce the problem.

Newcastle disease

This is caused by a highly infectious virus, with many strains of different virulence and tropism. The signs depend upon the strain of the field challenge virus. There may be an incubation period of 2–18 days, mostly at least 5 days.

The virus is transmitted rapidly from bird to bird by direct contact and via the air. This highlights the importance of good hygiene and site security.

Turkeys in general usually show fewer clinical signs of Newcastle disease than chickens although this does depend upon the strain of the virus, age of the bird, prior vaccination, environmental factors and the presence or absence of other diseases.

There is a sudden onset with many birds becoming listless and showing respiratory signs. High mortality may be seen in a young flock over a period of

5–6 days. If the birds are not eating, green bile-stained faecal droppings are present. Some birds will show nervous signs, especially bending the neck under or over the body, and paralysis; this is more common in younger birds. Breeders will show a reduction in quality and quantity of egg production, with increasing numbers of soft-shelled and misshapen eggs. Very mild strains of Newcastle disease virus may produce no signs or lesions whatsoever.

Any disease condition which does not respond to treatment should be investigated carefully for the possible presence of Newcastle disease in the background.

Gross lesions are dependent upon the strain of the virus. Some birds show large numbers of small petechial haemorrhages, especially on the heart, trachea, proventricular lining, mesentery and intestine. Others will show mainly respiratory tract lesions, and yet others mainly intestinal tract lesions.

Diagnosis is by isolation of the virus or demonstration of the increasing haemagglutination inhibition titre, which usually peaks at 7–12 days postinfection. There is of course no treatment other than helping the birds through the fever and treating any secondary infecting organisms that may be present.

Vaccination by using live vaccine in the fattening birds and a combination of live and dead vaccine in breeding birds is widely practised. Actual programmes depend upon the degree of field challenge in the area.

Ornithosis (Psittacosis Chlamydiosis)

This is caused by the Gram-negative organism *Chlamydia psittaci*, which has strains of varying virulence. Parrots and other psittacines, pigeons and gulls often have a latent form of infection and act as reservoirs. Ornithosis in turkeys is rare but it does occur and in some countries causes high mortality.

Ruffled feathers, inappetance and sometimes oedema of the face and coughing may be present. In some flocks there may be a severe fall in egg production. Some birds that have died show a fibrinous air sacculitis, pericarditis and peritonitis which is bacteriologically sterile on normal aerobic culture. Some birds may show congested lungs.

Diagnosis requires demonstration of the infecting organism. Treatment is by high levels of chlortetracycline for at least two weeks in the feed. Prevention is by excluding wild birds from all houses and ensuring all the usual hygiene precautions are followed.

Pasteurellosis (Fowl Cholera)

This is the most damaging bacterial disease of turkeys and can cause devastating levels of mortality. It is caused by the bacterium *Pasteurella multocida*, of which there are several different serotypes. It persists in the upper respiratory tract for long periods without causing any clinical disease but this may be precipitated by stress such as chilling, overcrowding, fighting, heavy ascarid infections and sometimes merely changes in the weather. Infection is passed from bird to bird or via the water or the feeders. Many survivors become carriers. The organisms are frequently introduced on the farms by rats and other vermin.

Good birds die suddenly, sometimes with bloodstained fluid oozing from their mouth and nostrils. In other cases they may separate from the remainder of the flock, looking rather dejected for a few hours before dying. A few birds may develop a chronic septic arthritis, when the joints will be filled with a pinkish necrotic material.

Gross lesions consist of a fevered carcase but the most common lesion is a severe pneumonia in which all the lungs or part of the lungs may be swollen and solidified with a dull pinkish 'cooked' appearance. When these lungs are cut they are quite solid and a sanguinous fluid oozes from the cut surface.

As with any septicaemic condition there may be a large number of petechial haemorrhages in the heart fat, gizzard serosa and mesentery. The liver may be swollen and congested and may be covered by yellow fibrinous deposits. In less acute cases there may be numerous small yellow foci scattered throughout the liver. Sometimes the disease is spread by AI procedures producing a very inflamed cloaca and uterus and purulent peritonitis but no lung involvement. All cases of yolk (egg) peritonitis should be checked bacteriologically for *Pasteurella multocida*. Diagnosis is based on the age of the birds, usually over 10 weeks, a rapidly increasing mortality and general appearance of the lesions. The suspicions may be confirmed bacteriologically.

Treatment is by use of the sulpha drugs (sulphaquinoxaline) or chlortetracycline in the water initially, followed by feed medication. Occasionally it may be necessary to inject a tetracycline.

Once the disease is brought under control the flock should be vaccinated if there is considerable time before slaughter. However, the vaccines available do not contain all the different serotypes. In general birds on problem sites and breeders are vaccinated twice.

Reticuloendotheliosis virus infection

This is the cause of one of the lymphoid leucotic diseases of turkeys. The virus is transmitted laterally and vertically. Infection is inapparent where adult birds are involved, but younger turkeys develop diarrhoea and leg weakness. Mortality can vary from zero to as high as 25%; more females than males die, which is unusual, and a resurgence of mortality occurs as breeders come into lay. The virus is immunosuppressive so the birds succumb to all the usual bacterial and fungal infections.

Gross lesions will depend upon the secondary infections but an enteritis involving lesions of *E. coli* septicaemia is often a feature. In older birds a striking feature is the liver, which is extremely enlarged and shows diffuse lymphoid infiltration. Nerve lesions are not present.

There is no treatment. Prevention is by ensuring that breeding stock are free from the infection; breeder replacement sites should have an all-in/all-out policy.

Salmonellosis

The genus *Salmonella* contains many species of bacteria, all of which may cause problems though some more than others. Two species, *S. pullorum* and *S. gallinarum* are generally restricted to poultry. *S. typhimurium*, *S. enteritidis* and *S. hadar* can cause high mortality, as can many other serotypes on occasion.

Salmonellosis is a septicaemia so the birds are disinclined to move, have ruffled feathers, look very dejected and die. Occasionally birds go blind following an infection or are lame due to a septic arthritis. This is more common in the cases of *S. pullorum* and *S. enteritidis* infection. Young birds are more susceptible than old, and stressed birds are more susceptible than unstressed birds. It is rare to see mortality in birds over three weeks of age.

Transmission is via the egg due to either direct transmission, in the case of *S. pullorum* and *S. gallinarum* or by contamination of the shells in the other cases. Therefore egg and hatchery hygiene are of primary importance. The birds may also become infected from the environment, food, personnel, vermin, etc.

Treatment is not usually advisable unless the mortality is high, when a drug to which the particular salmonella is sensitive is used. However, treatment tends to prolong the carrier stage, and it is impossible to eliminate salmonellae by the use of antibacterial drugs. In the UK all isolations of salmonella have to be reported to the Ministry of Agriculture, Fisheries and Food.

Staphylococcal infections

These are quite common as arthritic conditions. There is a chronic form known as bumble foot where the feet swell due to tracts of yellow pus throughout the foot. In other cases, especially after debeaking, staphylococcal arthritis can occur in the hock joints.

Staphylococci, *E. coli* and streptococci may all cause osteomyelitis, usually in the proximal head of the long bones. Treatment is usually ineffective.

Syngamiasis (gapes)

A small red parasitic nematode, *Syngamus trachea*, lives in the trachea of turkeys, pheasants and peacocks causing the condition known as gapes. It may be passed from bird to bird by ingestion of embryonating parasite eggs or infective larvae or indirectly through ingestion of earthworms, snails or slugs that contain encysted larvae. Once inside the bird, the maturing larvae migrate via the lungs to the trachea.

The birds become unthrifty and may die in severe outbreaks. So many worms may be present in the trachea that they will suffocate the birds. The birds breathe by throwing the head up, gaping and occasionally making moist snicking sounds. In heavy infestations, the worms can even be seen coming out of the mouth of the birds. The worms are obvious in the trachea, as a Y-shaped red object formed by the small male and much larger female being permanently attached for copulation.

Treatment is problematical; thiabendazole, mebendazole or tetramisole in the water have completely replaced the older traditional remedies. The advent of concrete floors in controlled-environment houses has gone a long way to eliminating this infestation, which can be a big problem when the birds are on pastures.

Turkey pox

This is caused by a virus transmitted by biting insects or via open wounds, especially associated with injuries caused by fighting turkeys. Mortality is usually low, unless the disease is complicated by other infections. During the viraemic stage, the birds are ill and may succumb to other diseases, especially histomoniasis.

Nodular skin lesions around the head are obvious. If there are no complications these wither and fall off in 3–4 weeks to remain as reservoirs of the infection in the environment. There is also a diphtheritic form in the digestive and respiratory tract which can cause wasting and impaired growth.

The whitish-yellow opaque elevated vesicles and nodules are seen on the non-feathered part of the body, often overlapping each other. They later form a crust-like grey or dark-brown scab. In the diphtheritic form, especially in stags, the lesions take the form of cheesy, necrotic diphtheritic lesions in the mouth and oesophagus. When removed, they leave bleeding erosions. Typical lesions are the easiest to diagnose. Atypical ones require histological procedures.

There is no specific treatment. All environmental stress and other diseases should be eliminated. Unaffected birds should be vaccinated. An all-in/all-out site regime with good interbatch cleanout and disinfection are essential for the disease to be eliminated.

Vaccines are very effective and are applied by plucking a few feathers from the inner aspect of the thigh and applying the vaccine with a small brush. Wing web administration should not be performed in turkeys, as this tends to lead to the development of pox lesions on the birds' faces when they sleep with their heads tucked under the wings. As with all vaccines, only healthy birds should be vaccinated.

Turkey rhinotracheitis

This is the latest viral condition to become a scourge in turkeys, spreading throughout Europe and Africa. It affects turkeys of any age. Spread is usually very rapid within a house and from house to house (though occasionally odd houses may be missed), and from site to site. The condition is caused by a pneumovirus.

The disease is a respiratory condition, varying from quite mild to extremely severe. Mortality, which may be up to 25% in severe cases, usually starts about a week after clinical signs are first observed, due to secondary bacterial infections. Breeding flocks show a massive drop in egg production, often with misshapen eggs, though production usually returns as quickly as it fell. The young birds may show oedema of the head, a catarrhal discharge of frothy mucoid material from the nostrils, which very quickly becomes blocked, and conjunctivitis.

On post-mortem very little is seen with the initial infection. Later, secondary infections cause bacterial septicaemias, with very moist serofibrinous pericarditis, perihepatitis, air sacculitis and often pneumonia. Tracheitis and rhinitis are also present.

There is, of course, no treatment for the virus but antibacterial treatment in anticipation of the secondary bacterial infections may be useful. However, sometimes there is no response. Adverse environmental conditions, such as overstocking and poor ventilation, tend to aggravate the problem.

A live vaccine is available in the UK, which is very effective on single-age sites but may lead to problems on some multi-age sites. The live vaccine available in France is milder and causes less vaccine reaction. It is administered by aerosol at 5–10 days of age. Inactivated vaccines to be used after priming with the live vaccine are available in some countries and are being developed in others.

Further reading

American Association of Avian Pathologists (1989) *Avian diseases manual* 3rd edn. Texas A & M University College Station, Texas.

Calnek B W (ed) (1991) *Diseases of poultry* 9th edn. Iowa State University Press/Wolfe Publishing (outside USA).

Jordan F T W (ed) (1990) *Poultry diseases* 3rd edn. Baillière Tindall, London.

Sainsbury D W B (1980) *Poultry health and management* 1st edn. Granada Publications.

Turkey production and health (1983) MAFF Reference Book 243, Reference Stationery Office, HMSO, London.

DISEASE PREVENTION AND CONTROL IN DUCKS

KEITH R GOODERHAM BVSc, MRCVS, DPMP

Introduction

The domestic rearing of ducks has been carried out for centuries in most parts of the world. Each country and each location has developed its particular form of husbandry. It is only in relatively recent times that attempts have been made to intensify methods of production. Whilst disease problems are considerable under traditional methods of production, intensification brings different problems demanding different preventive considerations.

Traditional husbandry methods vary from extensive rearing on natural water, on artificial ponds (Plate 13), on agricultural fields, whether grass or stubble, or in orchards. Sometimes production is in houses of varying degrees of openness to the ambient environment.

Intensive production uses controlled-environment housing in which growing ducklings are reared on wire mesh, slats, litter or a combination of these. Breeding stock as well as growers may be housed intensively or extensively. Husbandry methods may vary depending on whether the birds are meat-type breeders, growers or ducks reared for culinary egg production. As most intensive production is of meat-type breeding and growing ducks, reference will be made principally to the common problems encountered and ways in which their incidence or severity might be reduced. Where appropriate, references are made to problems particularly associated with the more traditional or more extensive production methods.

Breeding stock management

On the day of hatch ducklings destined to form a breeding flock will be treated differently.

Sexing

Ducklings are relatively easy to vent sex as the newly hatched male has a phallus some 3–4 mm long. Eversion of the vent reveals whether the bird is male or female. In untrained hands two problems have been seen. The first is rupture of the yolk sac due to excessive abdominal pressure. Mortality may sometimes follow within a day or two. Other birds will survive and grow normally.

The second condition seen in sexed birds is an increase in mortality due to 'starve-outs'. These are birds which die on or about the fifth day of age. They show no evidence of having eaten since hatching, having black changed bile throughout the intestine and a large gall-bladder. The incidence is different with different sexers. The actual cause has not been determined but control is effected by redeploying sexers who cause a high incidence of 'starve-outs'.

Identification

It is common to identify breeding stock or particular strains of stock by marking them in some way. Methods include wing-tagging, toe-slitting or toe-punching.

Wing-tagging

Wing-tagging involves the insertion into the wing-web of a pin-type or clip-type tag. The wing of the duckling is small and the wing web affords only some 2 mm of space. Even though correctly inserted, the pin-type tag can swivel over the end of the wing tip such that the muscles and bones of the wing pass through the loop of the tag. Growth of the bird and thus the wing can result in strangulation of the wing tip. It is necessary therefore to check manually every wing tag at about five days of age to ensure it is still in the same position. If it is not, it may simply be removed and reinserted correctly.

The danger with the tag clipped on with pliers is that the operator has no 'feel' for where the point is inserted. It may easily be clipped through muscle, or sometimes through the space between the radius and the ulna bones. With growth of the duckling the problem becomes severe, with infection also developing.

Such tags should never be used by untrained staff and should always be checked at about five days of age and removed if incorrectly placed. A new tag should be placed in the other wing, allowing the damaged wing to heal.

Toe-slitting

This is the cutting of one or more foot webs by means of a clean, sharp scalpel or scissors. Whilst the cut should be sufficiently large not to heal totally in later life, care should be taken to avoid cutting obviously visible blood vessels.

Toe-punching

Toe punching is the punching of a hole in the toe web. If this hole is too large it gets larger with increasing age such that it can become hooked on obstacles and can even tear. It is better to avoid such a means of identification, but if it is used and the hole enlarges, it should be cut to form a slit which will not then catch on obstacles.

Vaccination

Very few vaccinations are necessary in ducks, but one common disease controlled by vaccination is duck virus hepatitis (DVH).

Commonly the flocks of origin of the day-old ducklings have been vaccinated and thus confer passive immunity on their progeny. If this is not so and the day-old ducklings are to be placed on a farm where DVH is enzootic, then they should be vaccinated when day-old. DVH is a live viral vaccine administered via a stab through the foot web. It is important that birds receive the vaccine before coming into contact with the field virus. Because the vaccine virus is incompletely attenuated it will revert to pathogenicity when passed through the duckling. For this reason, the vaccine should never be used unless DVH is already present on the farm. Moreover, eradication of the disease from a farm cannot progress if the vaccine continues to be used.

Mixing of sexes

Imprinting is very strong in the duckling. It has long been documented that to ensure good fertility in breeding flocks, the birds should be reared together from the time of hatching onwards. However, this is not in fact necessary, and other aspects of rearing make it sometimes undesirable. What is important is that the males should not be reared as a single sex in isolation. They should be reared together with some females or within sight of females. Mixing the sexes should take place as soon as other management practices allow (say 12–13 weeks of age).

Brooding

As with brooding of other poultry species, the brooding of ducklings from day-old demands close attention to the birds' needs, particularly with respect to water, warmth, feed, ventilation, lack of competition and suitable housing.

Restricted feeding (Plate 14)

Over a relatively short period of time, meat-type ducks have been selected genetically for the traits of commercial interest. Initially this was growth rate, but subsequently aspects of carcase composition and feed conversion efficiency have become more important.

Increasing weight for age has led to reproductive performance, measured in terms of egg numbers per female and hatchability of eggs laid, being diminished. The performance may readily be recovered and indeed enhanced by restricting the growth rate of the parent birds. This is achieved by limiting the amount of feed given in order that a determined growth profile is followed throughout rearing. However, unless the restricted feeding is carried out correctly, problems of disease and mortality may arise.

Birds soon learn that feed is limited and eat as much as they can as quickly as possible when feed is given. The management aim is for each bird to consume its allocation of feed. For this to be achieved, numbers of birds in each pen should be limited and the feed must be well spread out. Failure to do this, in the first instance, leads to a wide spread of body weights. The next sign is that the males weigh the same or less than the females. This is followed by mortality of small emaciated birds, particularly males but also females. Tenosynovitis is a common finding in these poor birds. The lesions seen are of solid pus in the tendon sheaths of the legs, particularly of the hock region and those lateral to the head of the tibio-tarsus just below the stifle joint.

This problem can be prevented by ensuring that all the birds are grown as closely to the growth curve as possible. This means that the quantity and quality of food given must be adequate, that pellet quality is good and that the food is well spread.

To avoid the males suffering in the way described, they may be grown separately, either totally so or mixed with an equal number of females. It is important, however, to mix the sexes together as soon as the major risk period is over. This may be as late as 16 weeks of age. If left too long, mating during lay is inadequate and fertility of eggs is below optimum.

Another danger associated with restricted feeding is that of water availability. Because the birds eat as much feed as possible, the oesophagus is soon distended with dry pellets. As soon as the supply of feed has been consumed, the birds track to the water. If there is inadequate water supply, birds will pile up and some will easily die. This may be due to wet food being squashed up into the mouth so impeding breathing, or it may be that the food present at the entrance to the chest is pressed onto the syrinx by the weight of the other birds.

One thing is important: if water is not freely available due to poor water pressure or to water being frozen, food should not be given until the shortage has been corrected.

Restricted feeding results in lower mortality through the laying period. The details of this will be discussed later.

Rearing accommodation

Whilst it is necessary to provide indoor accommodation for the brooding period, many rearers move their birds to outside pens in fields, with, or usually without, access to inside pens or other shelter.

Outdoor rearing

Various problems arise associated entirely with the rearing of birds in open pens. These are related firstly to the weather and secondly to predators. Smothering can occur on the first or second night out of the brooders. If the temperature drops excessively during the night, birds will huddle together and some may suffocate. This is in fact less usual in birds on restricted feed than in growers fed ad lib. Prevention of this condition is by ensuring birds do not move outside until at least 3½ weeks old and by acclimatizing them to the temperatures which will be experienced.

Heavy rain, particularly on birds below five weeks of age, can result in chilling and even drowning. These birds are still inadequately feathered to resist such weather. Similarly, young birds still yellow with down and with very small wings cannot withstand hot sunshine. Older birds will cool themselves by standing upright and creating a breeze with their wings in addition to their whiteness reflecting much of the sun's heat.

Continuous wet weather may result in muddy pen conditions, causing much of the feed provided being unavailable to the birds. Additionally, wet muddy feathers result in greater heat loss from the birds, increasing the amount of feed used for maintenance. Adjustments in feed allocation are essential to see the birds through such periods. When mud dries on the feet and legs of ducks after a wet spell, it can be followed by the development of chronic infections.

The other weather hazards are frost and snow. Not only may birds be deprived of drinking water, but their feet and foot webs may become red and swollen. Care should be taken at these times to reassess the needs of the birds in terms of water, feed and shelter.

Predators are common when birds are reared in outside pens. Both birds and mammals will kill ducks. Birds such as gulls will pick out the weaker ducks and eat them while the duck is still alive. The main control measure in this instance is to remove the weaker birds from the flock as soon as they are detected and either cull them or put them indoors. Correct control of feeding and general stockmanship should reduce the incidence of weakly birds.

Foxes are important predators because they will kill large numbers of ducks, not just those required for food. Many of the ducks, having been chased around the pen, although not physically damaged will go lame. This 'psychological lameness' is common in ducks when they have been handled too severely. Domestic dogs will also kill or maul ducks. It is possible to distinguish between damage by foxes and dogs by the distance between the marks made by the teeth. If more than 2 cm apart a dog is involved. Other carnivorous animals will also prey on ducks if they are in the vicinity and can gain access to the duck pens.

Indoor rearing

Indoor rearing entails some of the problems encountered with outdoor rearing, plus some which are specifically 'inside' problems.

Stocking density is important because there must be adequate space for the feed to be spread and the litter must be maintained in a dry condition without excessive build-up of litter. Four birds per square metre is a maximum density.

The arrangement for drinking water should be such that birds do not panic for water after feeding but the drinkers should be sufficiently separated from the littered area to avoid excessive water being splashed or carried back onto the litter.

Fresh litter should be spread daily. This is usually either wood shavings or straw. Whichever is used it should be dry and of good quality. Straw in particular may be mouldy; it should never be used if it looks or smells mouldy. The inhalation of fungal spores will lead to fungal infection of the lungs and air sacs. This condition is usually called aspergillosis as the commonest infection is with *Aspergillus fumigatus*, but other species or genera of fungus are also seen which lead to respiratory distress and death in ducks. Prevention of aspergillosis not only involves avoiding the use of mouldy litter or other sources of mould (feed, old sacks, etc.), but the maintenance of good ventilation.

The laying period

A breeding flock may be brought into lay any time between 23 and 28 weeks of age. Much will depend on the strain of bird and the desired programme as well as the time of year. Ducks are brought into lay physiologically by increasing the daylength and by increasing their feed.

Feed is increased in quantity and quality, the diet being changed from a maintenance ration to a breeder ration. This sudden change can easily lead to mortality due to necrotic enteritis. Birds are found dead in good condition, usually in full lay. The carcase fat appears pinkish and greasy. Flakes of necrotic material are found in the terminal parts of the small intestine. This condition can be prevented by changing from maintenance to breeder diet whilst the quantity is still being restricted. Once accustomed to the new diet, the increase of feed and light may be started to bring birds into lay.

It is common to move birds from their rearing accommodation to their laying pens. This should be timed to take place before the birds start to lay, and the change of diet and increase in light should be programmed for after the move.

The stocking density in lay will depend on the quality of the housing, but should not exceed two females per square metre. (It is not usual to count the drakes when calculating stocking density.) Mating ratios are traditionally one drake to 4½ ducks. With restricted growth in rearing this should be widened to 1:6. With too many males, the incidence of damage caused by drakes in both females and males will increase.

Laying quarters

The quality and cleanliness of the hatching eggs determine the quality of the day-old ducklings. Nests must be introduced before the birds come into lay so that they learn to use them. There should be one nest for every five females. The nests should be on the floor, with a small (e.g. 10 cm; 4 in) front board, but should not be placed directly under the lights—ducks prefer to lay in a darkened area and will not use brightly lit nests. This tendency is exacerbated by not having lids on the nests to allow easier egg collection.

Even with an adequate number of nests, there will still be some favoured spots which are used for laying, typically in dark corners, by posts or at the end of a row of nests. These areas must be treated as nests when considering the hygiene of nests.

Nests should be littered with clean dry shavings, which must be replenished totally every week. The old litter may be used as part of the floor litter. Any bird droppings found in the nests in the meantime should be removed.

Egg collection is usually carried out once a day. The timing can be worked out by observation. Normal practice is for the lights to come on at 4.00 a.m. and for eggs to be collected between 7.00 and 7.30 a.m. It will be found that well over 90% of the daily production will be collected at this time, having been laid within the previous 3 to 4 hours. Collection should be onto plastic egg flats, not baskets, to avoid cracking. Dirty eggs and floor eggs should be collected separately. The daily littering of the pen floor should be done as late in the day as possible so that the conditions underfoot are clean and dry when the eggs are being laid. The litter used must be clean and dry, preferably wood shavings, although many people will use straw as it is more readily available. At the time of littering the pens, a second collection of eggs should be made.

The pen drinking arrangement should be well away from the littered area and nest boxes, preferably up a ramp on a mesh or slatted area. As long as there is enough watering space (about 1 cm (0.4 in) per bird) and the birds learn where it is before starting their reproductive tract development, then the watering area may be well hidden from the littered area. This will reduce the amount of water carried onto the litter.

Once the eggs have been collected it is important to wash them as soon as possible. Crucial factors when washing are temperature and time of wash, the sanitizing agent used and the number of eggs washed in a given volume of solution. This is a critical process, but the variations in programmes are considerable. Commonly, a chlorine-liberating sanitant is used at, say 40 °C (104 °F) for 5 minutes. Some iodophors are also useful. Dirty and floor eggs should always be kept separate and washed or sanitized last.

Vaccinations

There are few diseases for which breeding stock are vaccinated. Duck viral hepatitis has already been mentioned with reference to protection of the young breeders themselves. Important too, is the degree of protection conferred on their progeny. This is only important if the progeny are being placed on farms where duck viral hepatitis is enzootic. If the disease is not present on the growing farms there is no need to vaccinate. Where duck virus hepatitis is enzootic the planned programme would be two vaccinations (parenteral injection of live viral vaccine) prior to point of lay and another midway through lay. With this regime vaccination of progeny should be unnecessary.

Duck viral enteritis can occur in young ducklings as well as adults. Here, the vaccination programme is specifically to protect the laying flock. Vaccination using a live vaccine at 7 and 11 weeks, point of lay and every 4 months thereafter is the recommended programme. Vaccination is unnecessary unless the disease is likely to be present.

Pasteurella multocida can be responsible for heavy mortality due to an acute septicaemia in adult ducks. Whilst the disease is also seen in young growing ducks, it is particularly damaging to adult breeding flocks. The disease tends to have a history of occurring in certain areas and on certain farms. These farms are advised to pursue a preventive programme using a killed vaccine.

Diseases during lay

The most important diseases of the laying period are discussed below. Some of these have a lower incidence in flocks reared on a restricted growth rate than those fed ad lib during rearing. Indeed, the overall loss in the former group may be half that experienced in the latter group. Diseases which are influenced in this way are, particularly, amyloidosis, synovitis and other leg problems, and vent gleet (cloacitis).

Amyloidosis

This is a disease of uncertain aetiology in which amyloid tissue accumulates in various organs, particularly the liver. This results eventually in a grossly enlarged, hardened, sand-coloured liver, accompanied by an accumulation of ascitic fluid which distends the abdomen. The spleen is enlarged and haemorrhagic and may even rupture. A common finding is a vegetative endocarditis affecting one or more of the heart valves. This last lesion suggests that the disease has a chronic bacterial association.

Mortality from amyloidosis increases with age. Only rarely is it found in young growing birds where it is associated with chronic lesions of trauma. The incidence is high in heavy ducks, particularly elite genetic strains produced for maximum growth rate. Prevention therefore includes rearing on a slow-growth pattern. There is no treatment for the disease.

Synovitis (and/or Tenosynovitis)

This is seen affecting the legs of adult birds. The lesions of feet or hocks are chronic and large. Chronic indurated lumps of pus are often surrounded by fresh accumulations of fluid pus. These birds are usually quite heavy and have large calluses on the plantar pads of their feet. Amyloidosis may be a secondary feature.

This problem is again more common in birds reared to heavy weights. It is also more common in pen conditions where there is a high percentage of the floor covered by slats or wire mesh, particularly when these features become worn. There is no effective treatment for this condition, but it can be prevented by ensuring that all floors and equipment are in good repair and by rearing the ducks to a lower point of lay weight.

Vent gleet (cloacitis)

This condition is most commonly found in laying ducks. It is particularly associated with two factors—unhygienic conditions, particularly of drinking water, and the laying of large eggs. The size of the egg is less in flocks reared on a reduced growth curve and is less in birds fed a reduced level of feed in lay. This last practice requires close attention to the needs and behaviour of the flock if reduction in egg numbers is to be avoided. Ensuring that the heavy strains of duck do not lay eggs of more than 92 g (3¼ oz) will help to control vent gleet. It will also enhance the hatchability of the eggs laid.

Vent gleet is manifested as a semi-prolapse of the vent in some birds. When they are examined a yellowish plaque of pus is seen tightly adherent to the mucous membrane of the cloaca. The extent of these plaques will vary as will the number seen in any one vent. If the plaques are stripped off, the underlying congested tissues will haemorrhage. Treatment should be started early, as scar tissue will develop and reduce the ability of the bird to pass an egg. The next stage is difficulty in passing faeces or even a total healing over of the vent. Males are also seen to be affected and it is suggested that venereal transmission of the disease occurs.

Water troughs should be emptied and cleaned daily, and there should always be an adequate supply of fresh clean water available. Each bird should be allocated at least 1 cm (0.4 in) of water trough space.

Topical application of 1 ml of a 50 mg/ml suspension of furazolidone gently rubbed into the vent has been shown to be a useful treatment. In addition, plenty of fresh clean water medicated with a tetracycline results in improvement in the lesions. It would appear this is the result of topical application of the solution by the birds when preening. Stopping the birds laying will also reduce the incidence of vent gleet, but it does tend to recur in once-affected flocks when they are brought into a second lay.

Salpingitis

This is a condition seen in females of all ages, but which may cause a peak of mortality at point of lay. It is an occlusion of the oviduct to a greater or lesser part of its length with caseo-pus or solidified secretion from the oviduct. This has frequently been described as material of egg origin; whilst this may sometimes be so, it is by no means always true. Salpingitis at or about point of lay often results in the death of the birds, the ovary of which is only just developing in readiness for ovulation.

The original infection of salpingitis may occur as early as four or five weeks of age. It is one of the lesions associated with respiratory disease and septicaemia in the growing bird. Females experiencing this lesion may overcome the infection, but the now sterile pus remains as a foreign body. Such birds grow normally and are apparently healthy. For some reason, as the oviduct starts to develop, active infection starts up again, possibly from antiperistalsis from the cloaca. The developing oviduct secretes concentric layers of albumen-like material on the plug of pus. This all becomes inspissated. Active infection including peritonitis may ensue and death follows.

Sometimes the lesion does not become reinfected and the bird remains quite healthy, but becomes a blind layer, ovulating internally. Such birds can be identified on a trap-nesting programme. If healthy birds which have never laid an egg are killed and examined, this lesion may be found at post-mortem. Sometimes, however, the oviduct appears normal and is well developed. One or more clear, fluid-filled cysts in the ligament of the oviduct appear to prevent normal egg-laying and evidence of internal laying is found.

If flocks are reared on single-age all-in/all-out sites with good between-flock hygiene, the incidence of salpingitis at point of lay is greatly diminished.

Aspergillosis

As already mentioned this is a fungal infection of the respiratory tract (lungs and air sacs) resulting from the inhalation of airborne fungal spores. These may arise from mouldy litter, mouldy feed or some other dry mould source such as disturbed cobwebs and dust. Good ventilation helps to dilute any fungal spores within the atmosphere of the house. Some people will not use mouldy bales of hay or straw for litter but will use them as pen divisions. This is equally bad as the duck will 'dabble' into the depth of these bales.

The disease is chronic in adult birds. This is one disease which is purely managemental. As mentioned earlier, fungi other than *Aspergillus fumigatus* may be involved but they are similar in cause and effect.

Preferential mating

This is manifest in particular individuals as loss of feather on the back of the head and neck. The skin is reddened and even scabbed and weeping with serum. Subcutaneous oedema is common in this region. Such birds are eventually found dead. The lesion is caused by excessive mating by the drakes, and it may be found in males and females alike. An excessively close mating ratio of more than 20 drakes for every 100 ducks, may be the cause and the condition is indeed common where mature drakes are held together as a single sex. Preferential mating would be the primary diagnosis.

More commonly the excessive attention is directed towards an ailing bird, particularly if it is lame. A lame bird will sit for long periods and drakes behave as if the bird is 'crouching' for mating. In such cases 'preferential mating' would be secondary to the primary diagnosis.

Prevention is by ensuring the correct mating ratio, and by removing sick birds from the flock when they are first identified.

Prolapse of the oviduct

This is seen particularly in point-of-lay ducks which, as with other species of poultry, do lay a number of large double-yolked eggs. There is an increased incidence of prolapse associated with the production of large eggs from young birds. Affected birds are best culled from the flock. The problem may be reduced by ensuring the birds are not too fat at the point of lay.

Prolapse of the phallus

This occurs in the sexually mature male when the phallus instead of being retracted within the cloaca is seen hanging down from the vent. It becomes dirty and necrotic and the bird usually dies. The condition usually affects a number of drakes in the flock. Post-mortem examination frequently reveals infective material and reaction in the erectile tissue at the base of the phallus. It is this which prevents normal retraction. There appears to be no sensible treatment for affected birds. The problem may have its origins in an earlier septicaemic disease.

Hatching commercial ducklings

In the description of the parent day-old duckling it was assumed that it was a normal bird hatched from a normal egg. In describing the commercial day-old, disease conditions will be described which could equally occur in the parent or elite generation of day-old birds, therefore a day-old duckling may suffer similar disease irrespective of its genetic generation.

In describing the parent laying pens and nest boxes, considerable attention was directed towards aspects of clean, sound egg production and gentle handling. The reason for this is that many of the conditions which occur in the young duckling are the direct result of errors in these areas.

Egg-transmitted diseases

Whilst, inevitably, ovarian-transmitted infections occur, little description of their importance has been made. Diseases spread via the egg are the result of dirty egg shells and egg-shell penetration of organisms.

The normal egg, collected clean and fresh from a clean nest, will have a shell surface viable count of bacteria of one million or so. Benefit to both level of hatchability and viability of ducklings is achieved from egg sanitizing or egg washing. Merely fumigating with formaldehyde is not a successful approach. Washing of floor eggs and dirty eggs is of value, but hatchability and viability of the ducklings never approaches that achieved from clean eggs.

The first evidence of bacterial penetration of the egg shell during incubation is of eggs exploding in the incubators. This is due to the multiplication within the egg of gas-producing bacteria, causing a build-up of pressure sufficient to explode the shell. When this happens, infective material is splattered onto the shells of other incubating eggs, particularly those below the offending egg. Bacteria penetrate the unaffected eggs and start the process again. Seldom does an egg explode before the 13th day of incubation.

Prevention of this situation (other than the production of good-quality clean eggs) means firstly ensuring that any floor or dirty eggs are trayed separately and set on the bottom of the incubator shelves or trolley. Secondly, always candle eggs before the 13th day of incubation. Day 10 is ideal. Any stained-shelled eggs are again removed when the eggs are transferred to the hatchers on day 24 or 25 of incubation.

The details of good incubation are not given here (see Chapter 3) but suffice to say that only the correct approach results in the best-quality day-old ducklings. Incorrect incubation may lead to an uneven hatch with a number of 'late hatch' ducklings and dehydration of 'early hatch' ducklings.

Yolk sac infection

This is far more common in ducklings hatching from dirty eggs than from clean eggs. The bacteria involved in the infection may vary, but the most acute problems usually yield *Escherichia coli* on culture. Regardless of the organism, prevention is the same: attention to good hygiene of flocks, their housing, nests, eggs and hatchery.

Typhilitis (inflammation of the caecum)

This is a condition closely associated with yolk sac infection. When bacteria of low pathogenicity infect the yolk sac, they frequently infect the caecae also. Some strains of *E. coli* will do this as will some salmonellae (e.g. *Salmonella typhimurium*). In such cases, a peak of mortality is seen at 10–14 days of age.

Clinical signs are of dullness, head well pulled into the body, standing with a wide base but disinclined to move, wings drooped and the down harsh and staring. Birds are extremely dehydrated and eventually die. On post-mortem examination the caecae contain thin cream-coloured cores of pus. There is usually a medium-sized inspissated yolk sac. Urate nephrosis is a common finding. Bacterial culture will usually indicate which organism is involved. Sometimes multiple minute grey-coloured necrotic foci are seen throughout the substance of the liver. Some affected birds do not die, but the caecal walls become thickly fibrosed and the caecal cores enlarged and inspissated. Such birds do not grow well; they may eventually be culled or if slaughtered for meat are underweight, poorly fleshed and still show the chronic caecal lesions. The incidence of this condition is directly related to egg hygiene.

Aspergillosis

This has already been described as a disease of older birds. If pen and nest hygiene are not correct, fungal spores can get carried into the hatchery. Damp egg storage conditions may foster the growth of fungi before the eggs are set. More frequently, however, the ingress of the fungi into the egg is through hair cracks. In their turn, the hair cracks originate from poor egg handling. They can occur at any stage of handling but particularly hazardous is the collecting of eggs in buckets or baskets. Inevitably the weight of eggs on others will damage the shells and pressure occurs on all the eggs when the basket is lifted and the sides are drawn in. It is essential to collect onto egg flats, preferably in a holder in which each flat is on a separate shelf. If the flats are stacked on one another, there should always be a double thickness on the bottom to stop bending when they are lifted. The stacks should never be more than five flats high.

When the fungus does get into the egg it will grow during the incubation period and will kill the embryo. Frequently, however, the fungal growth occurs in the air cell, when it will sporulate. Opening this air cell other than very gently will release large numbers of spores into the air. If these are breathed in by the newly hatched ducklings, especially in the confined environment of a hatcher, then brooder pneumonia (aspergillosis) will rapidly develop. Affected birds will show a gasping or gaping respiration at the time of hatching or when they are placed in their brooding environment. These birds soon die and on post-mortem examination show multiple caseous nodules throughout the substance of the lungs.

The problem of aspergillosis can be avoided: good pen and nest hygiene, correct egg handling prior to and during incubation, avoidance of smashed candled-out eggs and hatch debris. Particularly dangerous is the non-pipped dead-in-shell category. If hatch debris is macerated within the hatchery, then these unpipped eggs should be removed before macerating the remainder. Alternatively the maceration should be done after the day-olds have been despatched and any aerosol generated should be ventilated out of the hatchery.

Over-fumigation

A common practice in hatcheries is to generate formaldehyde gas in the machines as the birds are hatching. If the concentration of this gas is excessive then it may cause damage to the respiratory tract. Affected birds show a gaping respiration similar to that seen in aspergillosis. The day-olds show a salmon-pink coloration of the down, making them look quite attractive compared with the yellow colour of the normal hatch. Birds showing respiratory signs will soon die. The lungs of these birds are virtually normal, the only lesion seen being a caseous plug at the opening of the larynx. Death is due to asphyxiation.

Brooding management

The basic requirements for brooding ducklings are similar to the requirements of other poultry species. These are the avoidance of chilling or overheating, the provision of adequate water and feed, and the avoidance of excessive competition. Protection from disease and predators is also important.

The physical structure and layout of the brooding facility may vary, with advantages and disadvantages for design. The most rewarding and successful brooding is achieved on plastic-covered wiremesh with wire centres no more than 2.0 cm (¾ in) apart. More open mesh causes walking difficulties, particularly for smaller or poorer quality day-olds. Such birds can be helped by having a close-mesh washable nylon net placed over the fitted wire for two or three days. There should be no draught from under the wire, nor should the area under the wire be cold. Ducklings like to be warm under their bodies when brooding.

Alternative systems have wire and litter or litter only. With wire and litter, the wire should be similar to that already described. The drinking water should be on the wire and ideally the ducklings should be confined to the wire area for the first few days depending on the stocking density there. The problem with an all-litter floor is that the more water provided the wetter the brooding conditions will be. This is not usually ideal if the birds are placed in large numbers (in excess of 100 birds per brooding population). It is better if the litter used is clean, dry wood-shavings rather than straw.

Heat may be whole-room heating or spot heating from infra-red electric bulbs or gas-fired canopy brooders. Using spot brooders allows easier provision of feed and water and enables the brooding population to be determined.

Considering the brooding population alone, when the feed and water space per bird is identical, competition starts to take effect when more than 400 birds are placed under a brooder. This has little detrimental effect until there are more than 600, especially when all aspects of room temperature, ventilation, feed and water quality, and positioning are considered. Exceeding that number leads to poorer growth, poorer uniformity and increased mortality and disease.

With spot brooding one has to consider under-the-brooder temperatures and room temperatures. The profile or reduction of temperature depends entirely on the age of move and the accommodation into which the birds will move. If they are to be placed in outside pens or semi-extensive unheated housing, then the ambient weather conditions must also be considered.

When placed as day-olds, the temperature under the brooder should be sufficiently high that birds do not want to sit directly under it, creating the typical 'O' shape of brooding recommended in the textbooks. The room temperature should be maintained at 28 °C (82 °F). Each day the room temperature is decreased by 0.5 °C, the brooder temperature decreased and the brooder height raised to maintain the O-shaped brooder ring.

Water must be plentiful in depth and in space per bird. If the day-old ducklings are dehydrated on arrival, once they have settled, are comfortable, warm and the room temperature achieved after the doors have been closed, they may be sprayed. A hand-held garden spray may be used, one which has a nozzle adjustable for a fine mist. The water used should be at room temperature, which can be achieved by filling the sprayer on the morning of delivery and leaving it in the brooder room. When spraying the birds, this fine mist is directed over their backs where it forms fine droplets. The ducklings should not be made wetter than this. About five seconds is long enough to spray 100 ducklings. It is better to repeat the operation after a few hours or on the following morning rather than make them too wet and cold on the first occasion.

The drinking-water space for day-olds must be at least 1.0 cm (0.4 in) per bird. The watering arrangement may comprise permanent troughs together with hand-filled supplementary drinkers. They must be placed sufficiently near to the brooders for easy access, must have an adequate depth of water and be set at a height for easy drinking. The design of the drinker should discourage the ducks from standing in the water. If supplementary drinkers are used they should never be allowed to run dry in the first 48 hours of life. To achieve this it is usually necessary to rinse out and replenish the water in these drinkers at least three times a day. If nipple drinkers are used, their supply of water must not be counted as contributing to the water space until the birds are seven days old and have been correctly weaned onto the nipple drinkers. The water pressure in these nipples is also important. They should be equipped with an open-ended sight line in which the water column should not exceed 20 cm (8 in).

A lack of available water, if marginal, will result merely in a failure of birds to grow adequately and evenly. Panicking for water may be seen around those drinkers which are present. The more severe consequences are extreme dehydration, white pasted vents and mortality. Post-mortem examination shows these birds to be underweight and severely dehydrated with visible deposits of urates in the kidneys and ureters. Many individuals have urates in the pericardial sac and possibly over other organs and in tissues and joints throughout the body. This condition is called visceral gout and when seen is an almost certain sign of water deprivation. Visceral gout may in fact be seen at any age, including adults, but under the conditions described here, mortality may occur between the ages of 3 and 7 days.

The other consideration at time of placing day-old ducklings is feed. Quality, physical form and availability are all important. Ducklings will eat pellets from day-old and in fact cannot eat adequately if supplied with meal or crumbed pellets. It is normal to scatter feed on sheets of paper or flat pans in order to create enough feeding space. This must be replenished regularly over the first few days. During this time, feed must also be in the permanent troughs in reasonably close proximity to the birds. Ducklings will be trained onto these before the temporary feed trays or papers are removed. There should be at least 0.5 cm (0.2 in) of trough space per bird.

'Starve out' is a condition which results in mortality at about five days of age. Birds die in a poor condition, very much underweight, usually lower than their hatch weight of 55 g. These birds have never eaten although this does not imply shortage of available feed. The cause is not known, although one occurrence is described with respect to young parent chicks (see page 240).

Chilling and overheating

These two conditions are a direct result of husbandry error. Correct setting and functioning of equipment is essential. More importantly, frequent visits to the young birds by an experienced stockperson will prevent any such errors and consequent loss of birds. As an absolute minimum, each brooder room should have three visits every day, each of at least 30 minutes duration, until the ducklings are a week old. Most problems at this age occur as a result of inadequate observation and attention.

Trauma and drowning

The commonest cause of trauma is foot trapping in the wire mesh. In the first two days of age, the toes of one foot are often trapped between the wire mesh and the underlying supporting structures. At about 14 days of age birds become trapped by the hock in mesh of 2.5 cm (1 in) square. Wings of young ducklings can similarly become trapped.

One form of large hanging plastic drinker has been associated with drowning at 10 days of age. It seems that the duck's body at this age fits into the trough tightly so that the bird cannot get out. Prevention of this problem is either by using plastic inserts for these troughs or to avoid their use until after two weeks of age.

Duck viral hepatitis

This should not be a problem in ducklings if the parents were adequately vaccinated. If this is in doubt, then day-old ducklings should be vaccinated before being placed under the brooders, using the live chicken egg-adapted vaccine by foot-web stabbing.

The grow-out facility

It is common practice, as already stated, to move birds from their brooding house or rooms into other accommodation either within the same house, in another house or into the open air. Numerous combinations of these alternatives exist, more frequently planned for economy of housing space than in the duck's best interest.

Some of the diseases which occur during the growing period are closely related to these moves and the husbandry provided. Close examination of the husbandry may help to decide which aspects or which details of management and husbandry are frequently associated with disease outbreaks. Preventive measures will then suggest themselves for future flocks of birds. In this way, eventually the best practice within a specific accommodation will be determined. In assessing the environment provided at any stage, one should consider temperature, ventilation, quality of air, cubic capacity of the building, floor space per bird, types of drinker and feeder and space per bird, floor type and litter quality, lighting and competition.

When birds are moved from one room to another it is usual to give them more space as they grow. Frequently this implies that they were reaching a crowded stocking density before the move. What happens under these circumstances is that the bird's body heat is difficult to dissipate by ventilation, especially if draughts are to be prevented. The room temperature may be controlled, but the temperature at bird level remains high as does the humidity.

To prevent disease problems, several steps should be considered:

1. Move birds earlier, at a time when the environment can still be controlled.
2. Always ensure the room receiving the birds is at a higher temperature (e.g. $+1\,°C$) than the room the birds are leaving.
3. Consider giving the birds only part of the new room for the first 24 hours, so that chilling will be reduced. This practice must not restrict feed or water space.
4. Try to avoid buildings with excessive cubic capacity. This mainly relates to roof height where space needs to be heated if problems are to be avoided.

All facilities provided must be in a good state of repair and the environment kept clean and tidy. If wire floors are not kept in good repair, birds will fall through them into the drainage pit where they will chill or drown. Sharp edges will cut feet leading to chronic infections especially of the leg joints. Poorly fitted floors may lead to foot and wing trapping.

Foreign objects are readily consumed by ducks. If these are sharp (nails, staples, etc.) they will penetrate the gizzards (traumatic ventriculitis) and result eventually in death. Pieces of string are similarly consumed and result in impaction of the gizzard and subsequently very poor growth.

When birds are moved the equipment in the new quarters is often different, to meet the needs of the larger birds. Close observation should be made to ensure it does not represent a hazard to the new birds. For example, wire floors can present a problem. Wire mesh of 2.5 cm (1 in) square will trap the hock and sometimes the wing of birds of about 14 days of age. The critical ages must be determined and preventive action taken. A sudden change on move, for instance from trough drinkers to nipple drinkers, must be avoided.

These above examples do not result in specific diseases, but nevertheless can be responsible for considerable losses.

If the particular move being undertaken is from an enclosed building to an open field, then proper acclimatization must be practised. It is not possible to provide artificial heat, but some form of shelter is advised for the first few nights. It is common for ducks of about three weeks of age to huddle at night and smother. This does not happen if the birds have been properly acclimatized.

Ducks older than about $3\frac{1}{2}$ weeks have a tendency to go lame when chased or moved. Special care must be taken when moving birds of this age or older to ensure that they are not driven hard or physically stressed in other ways.

Specific diseases of growing ducks

The specific diseases of growing ducks are considered below. They will not be described in detail, but particular attention will be given to precipitating factors and to available preventive measures.

Duck viral hepatitis (DVH)

This has been referred to with specific reference to vaccination. If inadequately protected, birds may succumb to the disease, usually in the first week of life, but possibly up to three weeks of age. This acute infection results in multiple haemorrhages throughout the substance of the liver. Otherwise birds are in good bodily condition and few other lesions are seen. Mortality levels may be high or very high. DVH may sometimes occur at ages greater than three weeks. On such occasions the disease is usually complicated by secondary bacterial infections.

Prevention of DVH is by vaccination, but in the face of disease passive immunity can be conferred by injecting ducklings with serum collected from recovered birds. This serum will contain antibodies to the virus. A better approach to prevention is by keeping the premises free from the virus. Good site security, good hygiene standards and single-age populations are all helpful in preventing the infection.

Astrovirus infection

This has been described as causing mortality in young ducklings. At one time it was thought to be a variant strain of DVH. It is particularly seen causing mortality with an associated fatty kidney lesion. It is frequently related to a move, often occurring a few days after moving ducklings from brooding facilities to intermediate rearing quarters. Correct acclimatization and handling during the move can be of great help in reducing the losses.

Pasteurella anatipestifer infection

This is a septicaemic disease caused by the bacterium *Pasteurella anatipestifer*, otherwise called *Moraxella anatipestifer*. Many serotypes of the organism are found, but few are associated with serious disease.

Incidence of the disease is closely related to husbandry and management. If outbreaks occur, detailed examination of all factors involved in rearing the ducks should be investigated. Of particular interest should be the temperature and ventilation provided. Good ventilation throughout the 24 hours of each day, but with the avoidance of draughts, is essential. Care in balancing the environments when moving birds cannot be stressed too heavily. Various inactivated vaccines have been made and used with some success. They are an adjunct to the good preventive husbandry described above, not an alternative to it.

When outbreaks of this disease occur, treatment with an appropriate antibacterial drug is of value. Best results are obtained when the antibacterials are given by injection. Streptomycin in combination with dihydrostreptomycin is useful, as is penicillin or any of the synthetic penicillins.

Pasteurella multocida

This has already been mentioned with respect to adult breeding ducks. Should it occur in young growing ducks the treatment is similar to that for *P. anatipestifer* infection (see above).

Escherichia coli.

This is found causing a septicaemic disease which in many respects is similar to that caused by *P. anatipestifer*. Prevention and treatment are along similar lines, although penicillin is ineffective.

Chlamydiosis (Ornithosis)

This may be found in ducks but it is not usually the primary cause of disease. The significance of any infection is the organism's ability to cause disease in humans. In this respect it is an important zoonosis.

Coccidiosis

Several species of coccidia have been isolated from both wild and domestic ducks. The one which can cause acute disease and mortality in domestic populations is *Tyzzeria perniciosa*. It is not common practice to include a preventive anticoccidial drug continuously in the feed. The incidence of the disease should be assessed, as should the circumstances under which it occurs. Preventive measures may then be applied. For example, in England the disease tends to occur in ducks in outdoor grass pens in the summer. On farms where this is the case, sulphaquinoxaline in the feed at an inclusion level of 250 mg/kg may be given. Other anticoccidials developed for chickens are sometimes toxic. The other preventive approach is to avoid the husbandry practices which allow the disease to occur. Should clinical infection be seen, therapy with a sulphonamide in the drinking water is effective; an interrupted medication regime is used.

Aspergillosis

Fungal infection of the respiratory tract, whether caused by *Aspergillus* species or other fungi, is very common in growing ducks. As has already been mentioned this is a direct result of mouldy litter, mouldy feed, other sources of fungal spores in the environment and/or poor ventilation. This disease may therefore be described as solely a problem of incorrect management. Prevention is by identification and correction of management errors. There is no sensible treatment available.

Mycotoxicosis

The growth of certain fungi on or in feed or feed ingredients often results in toxic metabolites of the fungi being present in the feed consumed by the ducks. Ducks are particularly susceptible to mycotoxins, which either cause mortality or result in varying degrees of suboptimal growth and feed conversion efficiency. Positive diagnosis may be difficult in other than extreme cases.

Good feed mill practice will always aim to minimize or prevent the use of feed ingredients of suboptimal quality (see Chapter 4). Good husbandry will ensure the correct handling, storage and use of feed when delivered. This is another disease purely related to management.

Other toxicoses

As with other livestock there is a wide range of materials which can cause poisoning in ducks. Some of these are more important than others because of the frequency with which they occur rather than the relative toxicity of the material concerned.

Anticoccidials

Some of the drugs which are commonly used in poultry medicine are not suitable for ducks (e.g. halofuginone, arprinocid, nitrofurazone). Toxicity from these is commonly caused by feeding ducks rations made specifically for other poultry species. This should not be done unless the feed contains no prophylactic or therapeutic medicaments. When medication is used in ducks it is frequently at a lower dose rate from that used in, for instance, the domestic fowl. Correct dose levels must be determined before use.

Rodent bait

This is a common cause of poisoning in ducks. Care must be taken to bait in sites to which the ducks cannot gain access.

Lead poisoning

This is very common in ducks, particularly those reared in a more natural environment. This condition is described below in relation to ducks with swimming water.

Ascites

This is similar to broiler ascites seen in growing chickens and is a condition in which fluid accumulates in the abdominal cavity. A precipitating factor may be a marginal level of mycotoxin.

Ammonia Blindness

Unless prevented from doing so, ducks splash water around the house so that the litter is usually quite wet. It is necessary where straw or wood shavings are in use to add fresh litter on a daily basis. Notwithstanding good drinker and litter management, levels of ammonia build up if the ventilation is inadequate. The first signs in the ducks are increased lacrimation and wet rings around the eyes. Encrustations then develop which frequently seal the eyelids together such that the birds cannot see. The application of antibiotic cream while prising apart the eyelids may be beneficial. Often the conjunctiva by this time has become opaque with scar tissue. No treatment can substitute for good preventive husbandry in not allowing ammonia levels to exceed 20 ppm at any time of the day or night.

High ammonia levels also increase the birds' susceptibility to respiratory infections. Quite commonly seen are swollen infraorbital sinuses, which may contain liquid or caseous pus. Organisms isolated are usually those associated with bacterial septicaemic disease (*Pasteurella anatipestifer* or *Escherichia coli*).

Tibial Dyschondroplasia

This disease is similar to that in broiler chickens to which reference should be made. It is particularly common in fast-growing strains of duck, but the birds may show no apparent signs. In extreme cases the tibio-tarsal bones enlarge and bow at their upper extremities and result in slow-growing, bow-legged ducklings. At present there is no sensible advice for reducing the incidence of this condition.

Rickets and Osteomyelitis

These are two other leg conditions which are grouped together not because they are related but, together with tibial dyschondroplasia and tenosynovitis, because they account for the bulk of the lameness seen in ducks.

The cause of rickets in fast-growing young ducks is not clear, but is probably not a primary nutritional problem. It is more likely to be a metabolic problem.

Osteomyelitis, particularly involving staphylococci, can frequently be found in growing ducklings. It is thought that the bacterium gains entry when various 'mutilations' are being carried out, such as debeaking (debilling), declawing, injecting, toe slitting or wing-tagging at day-old. Particular care, both hygienic and physical, is necessary when carrying out such operations. Beforehand, however, consideration should be given to deciding whether any such procedures are necessary. The Ministry of Agriculture, Fisheries and Food and the Agricultural Departments in Great Britain have published Codes of Recommendations for the welfare of livestock. The one relating to ducks recommends that in debilling no more than the downward projecting part of the bean of the bill be removed. Declawing is not recommended. Some other countries are more lenient in such matters.

Cannibalism

Ducks will under certain circumstances peck one another and draw blood. This is particularly so when new wing feathers are growing. In housed ducks some reduction in this can be achieved by dimming the lights. Searing the sharp part of the duck's bill can also help, particularly with the flightier strains such as Khaki Campbell.

Predators

Predators, whether carnivorous birds such as herring gulls and crows or mammals such as foxes or domestic dogs, will often kill or injure considerable numbers of ducks. Despite several scaring devices and physical deterrents such as electric fences, the surest way of preventing losses from predators is to keep the ducks permanently housed. If this is not possible, the problem can be largely prevented by keeping the ducks in protected enclosures or pens at night.

Rearing on water

Traditionally ducks have been reared on swimming water, and world-wide more commercial ducks are reared this way than are reared intensively. Access to swimming water allows a number of diseases to occur or enhances the possibility of others occurring. A wide range of parasites is found in such birds, often parasites with a water-borne intermediate host. Nematode worms, cestode worms, flukes and leeches are frequently present.

There are two situations which bring the parasitic burden to serious disease proportions. One is the heavy and continued overstocking of the water, the other is the introduction of young birds which meet a sudden challenge of infestations. The extent to which parasites will create a commercially damaging problem should be assessed for each situation separately.

The only sound preventive approach is to keep the ducks away from the water or to rear the ducks away from water until they are of an age to withstand the challenge. A major disadvantage with the use of swimming water is that such areas are attractive to wild birds, whether waterfowl or other species. Often these are migratory birds, and diseases such as duck viral enteritis or pasteurellosis can readily be introduced, as well as the parasitic diseases already mentioned. Chlamydia, salmonellae and influenza may also be introduced in this way.

Botulism

A common disease of ducks of all ages, most frequently associated with access to swimming water, is botulism. This is a fatal disease caused by ingestion of the toxin of *Clostridium botulinum*. This bacterium flourishes in rotting vegetation, particularly in warm weather. Vegetation which has been flooded and left to rot as the water receded, or aquatic vegetation exposed to rot as water levels drop are both likely sources of the bacterium. Ducks dabbling in this material ingest the toxin, which causes paralysis particularly of the neck muscles. Affected birds are often found drowned as they are unable to keep their heads out of the water.

There has been a report of fly larvae inhabiting this rotting vegetation or decaying carcases of birds or fish concentrating botulinum toxin in their bodies. Ducks eating these larvae can receive massive doses of the toxin. During hot weather, prevention of botulism is achieved either by keeping the ducks away from the water or by fencing off areas of rotting vegetation and removal of any carcases.

Lead poisoning

This has been mentioned earlier, but it has a particular incidence in ducks on swimming water if that water attracts anglers or wildfowlers. Anglers' lead weights or lead shot from gun cartridges are readily consumed by ducks. Prevention of this condition is either by denying hunters access to the area or by encouraging them to use lead substitutes for weights and shot.

Further reading

Calnek B W et al. (eds) (1990) *Diseases of poultry* 9th edn. Iowa State University Press, Ames, Iowa.

Friend M (ed) (1987) *Field guide to wildlife diseases vol. 1. General field procedures and diseases of migratory birds.* US Dept. of the Interior, Fish and Wildlife Service. Resource Publication 167. Washington DC.

Jordan F T W (ed) (1990) *Poultry diseases* 3rd edn. Baillière Tindall, London.

Ministry of Agriculture, Fisheries and Food (1987) *Codes of recommendation for the welfare of livestock:—ducks.* HMSO, London.

Sandhu T S A (1986) Important diseases of ducks. In Farrell D J, Stapleton P (eds) *Duck production science and world practice.* University of New England, Armidale, Australia, pp. 111–34.

Scott M L, Dean W F (1990) *Nutrition and management of ducks.* M L Scott of Ithaca, N.Y.

REFERENCES

Arafa A S, Bloomer R J, Wilson H R, Simpson C F, Harms R H (1981) Susceptibility of various poultry species to dietary aflatoxin. *British Poultry Science* 22: 431–6.

Bacon L D (1987) Influence of the major histocompatibility complex on disease resistance and productivity. *Poultry Science* 66: 802–11.

Bar A, Rosenberg J, Perlman R, Hurwitz S (1987) Field rickets in turkeys: relationship to vitamin D. *Poultry Science* 66: 68–72.

Bielorai R, Josif B, Neumark H, Alumot E (1982) Low nutritional value of feather meal protein for chicks. *Journal of Nutrition* 112: 249–54.

Bierne M J, Jensen L S (1981) Influence of high levels of pyridoxine on twisted legs in broilers. *Poultry Science* 60: 1026–9.

Briles W E, Stone H A, Cole R K (1977) Marek's disease: effects of B histocompatibility alloalleles in resistant and susceptible chicken lines. *Science* 195: 193–5.

Brue R N, Latshaw J D (1981) Growth and energy retention of broilers as affected by pelleting and by density of the feed. *Poultry Science* 60: 1630.

Buckle A E (1981) The occurrence of mycotoxins in barley stored on farms in England and Wales. *Proceedings ADAS Seminar on Mycotoxins in Animal Feedingstuffs, 25–26 March 1981.* Ministry of Agriculture, Fisheries and Food, pp 21–5.

Bumstead N, Huggins M B, Cook J K A (1989) Genetic differences in susceptibility to a mixture of avian infectious bronchitis virus and *Escherichia coli*. *British Poultry Science* 30: 39–48.

Calnek B W, Witter R L (1984) Marek's disease. In Hofstad M S (ed) *Diseases of poultry* 13th edn, ch. 16. Iowa State University Press, Ames, Iowa.

Charmley E, Greenhalgh J F D (1987) Nutritive value of three cultivars of triticale for sheep, pigs and poultry. *Animal Feed Science and Technology* 18: 19–35.

Cohen I, Hurwitz S, Bar A (1972) Acid-base balance and sodium to chloride ratio in diets of laying hens. *Journal of Nutrition* 102: 1–8.

Cole R K (1972) The genetics of resistance to Marek's disease. Oncogenesis and herpes viruses. *Lyon International Agency for Research on Cancer*: pp 123–28.

Cole R K, Hutt F B (1973) Selection and heterosis in Cornell white leghorns: a review with special consideration of interstrain hybrids. *Animal Breeding Abstracts* **41**: 103–18.

Couch J R, Craven W W, Elvenheim C A, Halpin J G (1948) *Anatomical Records* **100**: 29–48.

Crawford R D (ed) (1990) *Poultry breeding and genetics*. Elsevier, Amsterdam, New York.

Crittenden L B (1975) Two levels of genetic resistance to lymphoid leukosis. *Avian Diseases* **19**: 281–92.

Duff S R I, Hocking P M, Randall C J, MacKenzie G (1989) Head swelling of traumatic aetiology in broiler breeding fowl. *Veterinary Record* **125**: 133–4.

Edwards H M (1988) Effect of dietary calcium, phosphorus, chloride, and zeolite on the development of tibial dyschondroplasia. *Poultry Science* **67**: 1436–47.

Edwards H M, Sorenson P (1987) Effects of short fasts on the development of tibial dyschondroplasia in chickens. *Journal of Nutrition* **117**: 194–200.

Edwards H M, Veltmann J R (1983) The role of calcium and phosphorus in the etiology of tibial dyschondroplasia in young chicks. *Journal of Nutrition* **113**: 1568–75.

El-Boushy A R (1979) Available phosphorus in poultry performance of laying hens and their egg quality, hatchability, bone analysis and strength in relation to calcium and phosphorus in blood plasma. *Netherlands Journal of Agricultural Science* **27**: 176–82.

Escalona P, Pesti G M (1987) Research note: nutritive value of poultry by-product meal. *Poultry Science* **66**: 1067–70.

Fenwick G R, Curtis R F (1980) Rapeseed meal and its use in poultry diets. *Animal Feed Science and Technology* **5**: 255–98.

Gavora J S (1990) Disease genetics. In Crawford R D (ed) *Poultry breeding and genetics*. Elsevier, Amsterdam, New York, pp 805–46.

Gavora J S, Spencer J L (1979) Studies on genetic resistance to Marek's disease—a review. *Comparative Immunology, Microbiology, and Infectious Diseases* **2**: 359–71.

Gavora J S, Spencer J L, Gowe R S, Harris D L (1980) Lymphoid leukosis virus infection: effects on production and mortality and consequences in selection for high egg production. *Poultry Science* **59**: 2165–78.

Gilbert A B, Peddie J, Mitchell G G, Teague P W (1981) The egg-laying response of the domestic hen to variation in dietary calcium. *British Poultry Science* **22**: 537–48.

Greis C L, Scott M L (1972) The pathology of pyridoxine deficiency in chicks. *Journal of Nutrition* **102**: 1259–68.

Griffiths N M, Land D G, Hobson-Frohock A (1979) Trimethylamine and egg taint. *British Poultry Science* **20**: 555–8.

Grunder A A, Hollands K G, Gavora J S, Chambers J R, Cave N A G (1984) Degenerative myopathy of the musculus supracoracoideus and production traits in strains of meat-type chickens. *Poultry Science* **63**: 781–5.

Gyles N R (1989) Poultry, people and progress. *Poultry Science* **68**: 1–8.

Gyles N R, Brown C J, Whitfill C E, Johnson W A (1981) Heritabilities for regression and progression of Rous sarcoma in the chicken. *Poultry Science* **60**: 1663 (abs).

Hacking A, Rosser W R, Dervish M T (1976) Zearalenone-producing species of Fusarium on barley seed. *Annals of Applied Biology* **84**: 7–11.

Halley J T, Nelson T S, Kirby L K, Johnson Z B (1987) Effect of altering dietary mineral balance on growth, leg abnormalities, and blood base excess in broiler chicks. *Poultry Science* **66**: 1684–92.

Hamilton R M G, Hollands K G, Voisey P W, Grunder A A (1980) Relationship between egg shell quality and shell breakage and factors that affect shell breakage in the field. *World Poultry Science Journal*: 177–89.

Han I K, Choi Y J, Chu K S, Park H S (1988) The utilization of full fat soybean for egg production and egg quality in the laying hen. *Asian Australian Journal of Animal Science* **1**: 173–8.

Hanrahan T (1987). Antinutritional factors in feed ingredients. *Pig International* March: 40–1.

Harms R H, Damron B L, Wilson H R (1968) Performance of broiler breeder pullets as influenced by composition, of grower and layer diets. *British Poultry Science* **9**: 359–66.

Harms R H, Simpson C F (1975) Biotin deficiency as a possible cause of swelling and ulceration of foot pads. *Poultry Science* **54**: 1711–13.

Harms R H, Simpson C F (1977) Influence of wet litter and supplemental biotin on foot pad dermatitis in turkey poults. *Poultry Science* **56**: 2009–12.

Harper J A, Bernier P E, Helfer D H, Schmitz J A (1975) Degenerative myopathy of the deep pectoral muscle in the turkey. *Journal of Heredity* **66**: 362–6.

Hartmann W (1985) The effect of selection and genetic factors on resistance to disease in fowls—a review. *World's Poultry Science Journal* **41**: 20–35.

Hartmann W (1990) Evaluation of the potentials of new scientific developments for commercial poultry breeding. *Proceedings XIII European Poultry Congress, Barcelona, Spain* **1**: 156–64.

Haye U, Simons P C M (1978) Twisted legs in broilers. *British Poultry Science* **19**: 549–57.

Hesselman K, Elwinger K, Nillson M, Thomke S (1981) The effect of beta-glucanase supplementation, stage of ripeness and storage treatment of barley in diets fed to broiler chickens. *Poultry Science* **60**: 2664–71.

Hobson-Frohock A, Land D G, Griffiths N M, Curtis R F (1973) Egg taints: association with trimethylamine. *Nature* **243**: 304–5.

Hoerr F J, Carlton W W, Tuite J, Vesonder R F, Rohwedder W K et al. (1982a) Experimental Trichothecene mycotoxicosis produced by Fusarium sporotrichiella var. *Avian Pathology* **11**: 385–405.

Hoerr F J, Carlton W W, Yagen B, Joffe A Z (1982b) Mycotoxicosis produced in broiler chickens by multiple doses of either T-2 toxin or diacetoxyscirpenol. *Avian Pathology* **11**: 369–83.

Howell M V (1982) Moulds and Mycotoxins in Animal Feedstuffs. In Wiseman W (ed) *Recent Advances in Animal Nutrition*. Butterworths, London, pp 3–20.

Hulan H W, De Groote G, Fontaine G, De Munter G, McRae K B et al. (1986) Effects of different totals and ratios of dietary calcium and phosphorus on the performance and incidence of leg abnormalities in male broiler chickens derived from normal and dwarf maternal genotypes. *Canadian Journal of Animal Science* **66**: 167–79.

Hulan H W, Proudfoot F G, Ramey D, McRae K B (1980) Influence of genotype and diet on general performance and incidence of leg abnormalities of commercial broilers reared to roaster weights. *Poultry Science* **59**: 748–57.

Hulan H W, Simons P C M, Van Schagen P J W, McRae K B, Proudfoot F G (1987). Effect of dietary cation-anion balance and calcium content on general performance and incidence of leg abnormalities of broiler chickens. *Canadian Journal of Animal Science* **67**: 165–77.

Hurwitz S, Bar A, Meshorer A (1973). Field rickets in turkey poults: field observations and pathological, radiological and serological findings. *Poultry Science* **61**: 1370–74.

Hutt F B (1958) *Genetic resistance to disease in domestic animals*. Comstock Publishing Associates, Ithaca, New York.

Itakura C, Hakotani Y, Goto M, Saito T, Ishii K (1981) Histopathology of gizzard erosion in young broiler chickens due to fish meal in the diet. *Japanese Journal of Veterinary Science* **43**(5): 677–87.

Jackson S, Summers J D, Leeson S (1982) Effect of dietary protein and energy on broiler performance and production costs. *Poultry Science* **61**: 2232–40.

Jensen L S, Martinson R M, Schumaier G (1970) A foot pad dermatitis in turkey poults associated with soybean meal. *Poultry Science* **49**: 76–82.

Jeroch H (1987) Nutritional value of wheat, rye and triticale in broiler chickens and laying hens. *Proceedings of the 6th European Symposium on Poultry Nutrition*, October 1987. Königslutter FR Germany: A4–A14. World Poultry Science Association.

Jones J F, Hughes B L, Barnet B D (1976) Effect of feed regimes on body weight of turkey hens at 32 weeks of age and subsequent reproductive performance. *Poultry Science* **55**: 1356–60.

Julian R J (1990a) Musculo-skeletal disease in poultry: an overview of current problems. In *Avian skeletal disease symposium AAAP/AVMA, July 1990, AAAP/AVMA, San Antonio, Texas, pp 1–11.*

Julian R J (1990b) Pulmonary hypertension: a cause of right heart failure, ascites in meat-type chickens. *Feedstuffs* (29 January 1990) **62**(5): 19–22.

Julian R J (1990c) Influence of genetics on right heart failure and ascites in poultry caused by the pulmonary hypertension syndrome. In *Proceedings National Breeders' Roundtable, May 1990, St. Louis, Missouri.* Poultry Breeders of America, Atlanta, Georgia.

Karunajeewa H, Tham S H, Abuserewa S (1989) Sunflower seed meal, sunflower oil and full fat sunflower seeds, hulls and kernels for laying hens. *Animal Feed Science and Technology* **26**: 45–54.

Krogdahl A (1985) Digestion and absorption of lipids in poultry. *Journal of Nutrition* **115**: 675–85.

Krueger K K, Owen J A, Krueger C E, Ferguson T M (1978) Effect of feed and light regimes during the growing period on subsequent reproductive performance of broad breasted white turkeys fed two protein levels. *Poultry Science* **57**: 27–37.

Kuhnlein V, Sabour M, Gavora J S, Fairfull R W, Bernon D E (1989) Influence of selection for egg production and Marek's disease resistance on the incidence of endogenous viral genes in white leghorns. *Poultry Science* **68**: 1161–7.

Leach R M, Nesheim M C (1965) Nutritional, genetic and morphological studies of an abnormal cartilage formation in young chicks. *Journal of Nutrition* **86**: 236–44.

Leeson S, Summers J D (1988) Some nutritional implications of leg problems with poultry. *British Journal of Nutrition* **144**: 81–92.

Luckham D G, Slinger S J, Sibbald I R, Ashton G C (1963) Methods of restricting feed or energy intake of growing leghorn pullets and their effects on subsequent reproductive performance. *Poultry Science* **42**: 1285.

Mangan J L (1988) Nutritional effects of tannins in animal feeds. *Nutrition Research Reviews* **1**: 209–31.

Marks H L (1985) Sexual dimorphism in early feed and water intake of broilers. *Poultry Science* **64**: 425–8.

Martland M F (1985) Ulcerative dermatitis in broiler chickens: the effects of wet litter. *Avian Pathology* **14**: 353–64.

Masumura T, Sugahara M, Noguchi T, Mori K, Naito H (1985) The effect of gizzerosine, a recently discovered compound in over-heated fish meal, on the gastric acid secretion in chicken. *Poultry Science* **64**: 356–61.

McNaughton J L, Reece F N (1982) Influence of dietary energy on the effectiveness of pelleting. *Poultry Science* **61**: 1389.

McNulty M S, Connor T J, McNeilly F, Kirkpatrick K S, McFerran J B (1988) A serological survey of domestic poultry in the United Kingdom for antibody to chicken anaemia agent. *Avian Pathology* **17**: 315–24.

Miles R O (1981) Electrolytes and egg shell quality. *Proceedings Arkansas Nutrition Conference*. Arkansas Feed Manufacturer's Association and Department of Animal Science, University of Arkansas.

Miles R D, Costa P T, Harms R H (1983) The influence of dietary phosphorus level on laying hen performance, egg shell quality and various blood parameters. *Poultry Science* **62**: 1033-7.

Miles R D, Harms R H (1982) Relationship between egg specific gravity and plasma phosphorus from hens fed different dietary calcium, phosphorus and sodium levels. *Poultry Science* **61**: 175-7.

Mongin P (1968) Role of acid-base balance in the physiology of eggshell formation. *World Poultry Science Journal* **24**: 300-30.

Mongin P (1980a) Roles of sodium, potassium and chloride in eggshell quality. *Proceedings of the Florida Nutrition Conference*, Gainesville, Florida, pp 213-23.

Mongin P (1980b) Electrolytes in nutrition application in poultry and swine. *Proceedings of the Third Minerals Conference*, pp 1-15.

Nelson T S, Kirby L K, Johnson Z B, Beasley J N (1981) Effect of altering the dietary cation and anion content with magnesium and phosphorus on chick performance. *Poultry Science* **60**: 1030-5.

Newcombe M, Summers J D (1984) Effect of previous diet on feed intake and body weight gain of broiler and leghorn chicks. *Poultry Science* **63**: 1237-42.

Nixey C (1989) Nutritional responses of growing turkeys. In Nixey C, Grey T C (eds) *Recent Advances in Turkey Science. Proc 21st WPSA Poultry Science Symposium, September 1987*. Butterworth, London, pp 183-99.

Olson W G, Dzuik H, Walser M, Hanlon G F, Waibel P E et al. (1981) Field rickets in turkey poults: biochemical findings. *Avian Diseases* **25**: 550-4.

Pattison M, Chettle N, Randall C J, Wyeth P J (1989) Observations on swollen head syndrome in broiler and broiler breeder chickens. *Veterinary Record* **125**: 229-31.

Pesti G M, Smith C F (1984) The response of growing broiler chickens to dietary contents of protein, energy and added fat. *British Poultry Science* **25**: 127-38.

Potter L M, Leighton A T (1973) Effect of diet and light during the pre-breeder period and of the diet during the breeder period on turkey breeder performance. *Poultry Science* **52**: 1805-13.

Pustai A (1989) Antinutrients in rapeseeds. *Nutrition Abstracts and Reviews* **59**: 427-33.

Roland D A, Farmer M (1986) Studies concerning possible explanations for the varying response of different phosphorus levels on egg shell quality. *Poultry Science* **65**: 956-963.

Rudgren M (1988) Evaluation of triticale given to pigs, poultry and rats. *Animal Feed Science and Technology* **19**: 359-75.

Ruiz N, Harms R H, Linda S B (1990) Niacin Requirement of Broiler Chickens Fed a Corn-Soybean Meal Diet from 1 to 21 days of age. *Poultry Science* **69**: 433-9.

Sauveur B, Mongin P (1978) Tibial dyschondroplasia, a cartilage abnormality in poultry. *Annals Biology Animal Biochemistry and Biophysics* **18**: 87-98.

Singsen E P, Nagel J, Patrick S G, Matterson L D (1964) The effect of a lysine deficiency on body weight and age at sexual maturity. *Poultry Science* **43**: 786-7.

Siller W G (1985) Deep pectoral myopathy: a penalty of successful selection for muscle growth. *Poultry Science* **64**: 1591-5.

Slominski B A, Campbell L D, Stanger N E (1988) Extent of hydrolysis in the intestinal tract and potential absorption of intact glucosinolates in laying hens. *Journal Science Food Agriculture* 42: 305–14.

Spackman D (1985) The effect of disease on egg quality. In Wells R G, Belyavin C G (eds) *Egg quality: current problems and recent advances.* Butterworths, London.

Struthers B J, MacDonald J R (1983) Comparative inhibition of trypsins from several species by soybean by soybean trypsin inhibitors. *Journal of Nutrition* 113: 800–4.

Szylit O, Durand M, Borgida L P, Atinkpahoun H, Frieto F et al. (1978) Raw and steam pelleted cassava, sweet potato and yam cayenensis as starch sources for ruminant and chicken diets. *Animal Feed Science and Technology* 3: 73–8.

Tabib Z, Jones F T, Hamilton P B (1984) Effect of pelleting of poultry feed on the activity of moulds and mould inhibitors. *Poultry Science* 63: 70–5.

The Poultry Laying Flocks (Testing and Registration) Order 1989.

The Poultry Breeding Flocks and Hatcheries (Registration and Testing) Order 1989.

Touchburn S D, Naber E C, Chamberlin V D (1968) Effect of growth restriction on reproductive performance of turkeys. *Poultry Science* 47: 547–56.

Tung H T, Smith J W, Hamilton P B (1971) Aflatoxicosis and bruising in the chicken. *Poultry Science* 50: 793.

Vaughters P D, Pesti G M, Howarth B (1987) Effects of feed composition and feeding schedule on growth and development of broiler breeder males. *Poultry Science* 66: 134–46.

Voitle R A, Wilson H R, Harms R H (1974) Comparison of various methods of nutrient restriction for delaying sexual maturity in broiler breeder hens. *Nutrition Reports International* 9: 149–57.

Wakeling D E (1982) A fishy taint in eggs: Interaction between fishmeal diets and strain of bird. *British Poultry Science* 23: 89–93.

Waldroup P W, Damron B L, Harms R H (1966) The effect of low protein and high fiber grower diets on the performance of broiler pullets. *Poultry Science* 45: 393–401.

Walser M M, Hanlon G F, Newman J A, Dzuik H E, Olsen W G et al. (1980) Field rickets in turkey poults: field observations and pathological, radiological and serological findings. *Avian Diseases* 24: 309–16.

Washburn K W (1982) Incidence, cause, and prevention of egg shell breakage in commercial production. *Poultry Science* 61: 2005–12.

Wessela J P H, Post B J (1989) Effect of heat treatment of fish meals, fines and the addition of lysine as related to gizzard erosion in chickens. *Journal Science Food and Agriculture* 46: 393–406.

Whitehead C C (1989) Nutrition of turkey breeding stock. In Nixey C, Grey T C (eds) *Recent Advances in Turkey Science. Proc 21st WPSA Poultry Science Symposium, September 1987.* Butterworth, London, pp 91–117.

Whitehead C C, Blair R (1974) The involvement of biotin in the fatty liver and kidney syndrome in broiler chickens. *World Poultry Science Journal* 30: 231.

Whitehead C C, Blair R, Bannister D W, Evans A J (1975) The involvement of dietary fat and vitamins, stress, litter and starvation on the incidence of the fatty liver and kidney syndrome in broiler chickens. *Research in Veterinary Science* 18: 100–104.

Wilson J L, McDaniel G R, Sutton C D (1987) Dietary protein levels for broiler breeder males. *Poultry Science* 66: 237–42.

Wong-Valle J, McDaniel R G, Bartels J E, Kuhlers D L (1990) Incidence of tibial dyschondroplasia in broiler breeders after two generations of selection. *Poultry Science* **69** (Supp): 145 (abs).

Wyatt R D, Doerr J A, Hamilton P B, Burmeister H R (1975) Egg production, shell thickness, and other physiological parameters of laying hens affected by T-2 toxin. *Applied Microbiology* **29**: 641–45.

Wyeth P J, Chettle N, Gough R E, Collings M S (1987) Antibodies to TRT in chickens with swollen head syndrome. *Veterinary Record* **120**: 286–7.

INDEX

CPSIA information can be obtained
at www.ICGtesting.com
Printed in the USA
JSHW030018200821
17905JS00001B/22